The Comprehensive Cancer Center

Mahmoud Aljurf • Navneet S. Majhail
Mickey B. C. Koh
Mohamed A. Kharfan-Dabaja • Nelson J. Chao
Editors

The Comprehensive Cancer Center

Development, Integration,
and Implementation

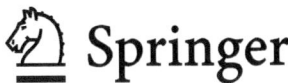 Springer

Editors
Mahmoud Aljurf
Oncology Centre
King Faisal Specialist Hosp and Res Ctr
Riyadh
Saudi Arabia

Mickey B. C. Koh
Stem Cell Transplantation
St George's, University of London
London
UK

Nelson J. Chao
Hematologic Malignancies and
Cellular Therapy
Duke University
Durham, NC
USA

Navneet S. Majhail
Blood and Marrow Transplant Program
Cleveland Clinic
Cleveland, OH
USA

Mohamed A. Kharfan-Dabaja
Blood and Marrow Transplantation
Mayo Clinic
Jacksonville, FL
USA

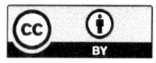

This book is an open access publication.

ISBN 978-3-030-82051-0   ISBN 978-3-030-82052-7   (eBook)
https://doi.org/10.1007/978-3-030-82052-7

This Springer imprint is published by the registered company Springer Nature Switzerland AG
The registered company address is: Gewerbestrasse 11, 6330 Cham, Switzerland

Contents

Contributors

Jame Abraham, MD, FACP Department of Hematology-Oncology, Cleveland Clinic Taussig Cancer Center, Cleveland, OH, USA

Gabriel Alcantara, MBA Duke Cancer Institute, Duke University Department of Medicine, Division of Hematologic Malignancies & Cellular Therapy, Durham, NC, USA

Mohamed Aldehaim, MD Department of Radiation Oncology, King Faisal Specialist Hospital & Research Center, Riyadh, Saudi Arabia

Saud Alhayli, MD Oncology Center, King Faisal Specialist Hospital & Research Centre, Riyadh, Saudi Arabia

Mahmoud Aljurf, MD Adult Hematology and HSCT, Oncology Centre, King Faisal Specialist Hospital & Research Centre, Riyadh, Saudi Arabia

Oncology Center, King Faisal Specialist Hospital & Research Centre, Riyadh, Saudi Arabia

Arslan Babar, MD Taussig Cancer Institute, Cleveland Clinic Foundation, Cleveland, OH, USA

Rajshekhar Chakraborty, MD Columbia University Medical Center, New York, NY, USA

Nelson J. Chao, MD, MBA Division of Hematologic Malignancies and Cellular Therapy/BMT, Global Cancer/Duke Cancer Institute/Duke Global Health Institute, Durham, NC, USA

Lita Chew, BCOP, FPSS Pharmacy, National Cancer Centre Singapore, Singapore, Singapore

Singapore Health Services, Singapore, Singapore

Department of Pharmacy, National University of Singapore, Singapore, Singapore

Chief Pharmacist Office, Ministry of Health, Singapore, Singapore

Singapore Pharmacy Council, Singapore, Singapore

Marcos De Lima, MD Blood and Marrow Transplant and Cellular Therapy, Ohio State University, Columbus, OH, USA

Kathryn M. Fleming, MD Department of Haematology, St Georges University Hospital, London, UK

Jennifer Frith, MSN, RN, OCN, NE-BC Inpatient Oncology and ABMT, Durham, NC, USA

Fady Geara, MD Naef K. Basile Cancer Institute, Department of Radiation Oncology, American University of Beirut, Beirut, Lebanon

Usama Gergis, MD, MBA Medical Oncology, Thomas Jefferson University Hospital, Philadelphia, PA, USA

Dolores Grosso, DNP, CRNP Medical Oncology, Thomas Jefferson University Hospital, Philadelphia, PA, USA

Shahrukh K. Hashmi, MD, MPH Division of Hematology, Department of Medicine, Mayo Clinic, Rochester, MN, USA

Sheikh Shakhbout Medical City, Abu Dhabi, UAE

Fazal Hussain, MD, MPH College of Medicine, Alfaisal University, Riyadh, Saudi Arabia

Mohamed A. Kharfan-Dabaja, MD, MBA Division of Hematology-Oncology and Blood and Marrow Transplantation Program, Mayo Clinic, Jacksonville, FL, USA

Blood and Marrow Transplantation Program, Mayo Clinic, Jacksonville, FL, USA

Matthias Klammer, MD Department of Haematology, St Georges University Hospital, London, UK

Liang Piu Koh, MD Department of Hematology-Oncology, National University Cancer Institute, National University Health System, Singapore, Singapore

Mickey B. C. Koh, MD, PhD Department of Haematology, St George's University Hospital, London, UK

Stem Cell Transplantation, Institute of Infection and Immunity, St George's Medical School, University of London, London, UK

Cell Therapy Facility, Health Sciences Authority, Singapore, Singapore

Francesca Lorraine Wei Inng Lim, MD Department of Hematology, Singapore General Hospital, SingHealth, Singapore, Singapore

Navneet S. Majhail, MD, MS Blood and Marrow Transplant Program, Department of Hematology-Oncology, Cleveland Clinic Taussig Cancer Center, Cleveland, OH, USA

Blood and Marrow Transplant Program, Cleveland Clinic, Cleveland, OH, USA

Rami Manochakian, MD Division of Hematology-Oncology, Mayo Clinic, Jacksonville, FL, USA

Asem Mansour, MD King Hussein Cancer Center, Amman, Jordan

Susan McInnes, MD Department of Palliative & Supportive Care, Taussig Cancer Institute, Cleveland Clinic, Cleveland, OH, USA

Miko Chui Mei Thum, BCOP, BCPS Chief Pharmacist Office, Ministry of Health, Singapore, Singapore

National Cancer Centre Singapore, Singapore, Singapore

Alberto J. Montero, MD, MBA Breast Cancer Program, UH Seidman Cancer Center, Diana Hyland Chair for Breast Cancer, Cleveland, OH, USA

CWRU School of Medicine, Cleveland, OH, USA

Hemant S. Murthy, MD Division of Hematology-Oncology, Mayo Clinic, Jacksonville, FL, USA

Blood and Marrow Transplantation Program, Mayo Clinic, Jacksonville, FL, USA

Jack Phan, MD, PhD Department of Radiation Oncology, The University of Texas MD Anderson Cancer Center, Houston, TX, USA

Laura Shoemaker, DO Department of Palliative & Supportive Care, Taussig Cancer Institute, Cleveland Clinic, Cleveland, OH, USA

Ian Qianhuang Wu, MD Department of Hematology-Oncology, National University Cancer Institute, National University Health System, Singapore, Singapore

Farah Yassine, MD, MS Division of Hematology-Oncology and Blood and Marrow Transplantation Program, Mayo Clinic, Jacksonville, FL, USA

Chapter 1
Introduction

Mahmoud Aljurf, Navneet S. Majhail, Mickey B. C. Koh, Mohamed A. Kharfan-Dabaja, and Nelson J. Chao

Cancer is a growing healthcare problem worldwide with significant public health and economic burden to both developed and developing countries. According to the World Health Organization, cancer is the second leading cause of death globally, with an estimated 20 million new cancer cases and 10 million cancer deaths in 2020. The International Agency for Cancer Research (IARC) estimates that globally one in five people will develop cancer in their lifetime. Low- and middle-income countries have been disproportionately affected by the rise of cancer incidence and account for approximately 70% of global cancer deaths. At the same time, substantial innovations in screening, diagnosis, and treatment of cancer have improved patient outcomes; global age-standardized cancer death rates showed a 17% decline from 1990 to 2016.

M. Aljurf (✉)
Adult Hematology and HSCT, Oncology Centre, King Faisal Specialist Hospital & Research Centre, Riyadh, Saudi Arabia
e-mail: maljurf@kfshrc.edu.sa

N. S. Majhail
Blood and Marrow Transplant Program, Department of Hematology-Oncology, Cleveland Clinic Taussig Cancer Center, Cleveland, OH, USA

M. B. C. Koh
Department of Haematology, St George's University Hospital, London, UK

Stem Cell Transplantation, Institute of Infection and Immunity, St George's Medical School, University of London, London, UK

Cell Therapy Facility, Health Sciences Authority, Singapore, Singapore

M. A. Kharfan-Dabaja
Division of Hematology-Oncology, Mayo Clinic, Jacksonville, FL, USA

Blood and Marrow Transplantation Program, Mayo Clinic, Jacksonville, FL, USA

N. J. Chao
Division of Hematologic Malignancies and Cellular Therapy/BMT, Global Cancer/Duke Cancer Institute/Duke Global Health Institute, Durham, NC, USA

M. Aljurf et al. (eds.), *The Comprehensive Cancer Center*,
https://doi.org/10.1007/978-3-030-82052-7_1

1

Cancer care has evolved to become highly specialized and increasingly complex not only pertaining to care setup and delivery, but also diagnostics and therapeutics. In addition, the influx of novel therapies such as targeted therapy, biologics, cellular and gene therapies, the need for advanced support systems such as advanced pathology, radiology, and radiation therapy, and the requirement for integrated multidisciplinary delivery of care had contributed to the progressive increase in the costs of cancer care both direct expenditures related to infrastructure and provision of care from a societal perspective, as well as indirect costs due to loss of productivity at an individual level. Presently, many hospitals and cancer centers may not have a well-established and integrated setup for comprehensive and cost-effective oncology care.

The objective of this book is to provide guidance to hospitals, institutions, and health authorities worldwide to develop a comprehensive cancer care plan; and to assist cancer centers with upgrading their existing infrastructure, practice standards, policies, and procedures in line with contemporary and highest international standards for cancer care delivery, in a sustainable and cost-effective manner.

Each chapter tackles an aspect felt by the editors to be critical in the design of such centers especially as these are developed in low- to middle-income countries. The contents of this book are applicable at a global level and do cover broad aspects related to the overall organizational structure of a comprehensive cancer center, including inpatient and outpatient services, pharmacy and laboratory requirements, radiation therapy, psychosocial support and palliative care, among others. The book also covers staff training, quality and data management, and overall administration including finance and strategic planning. One chapter is specifically dedicated to cancer management for a center with restricted resources.

Inequality and disparities in healthcare between higher and lower resource settings is well known. The authors and the editors hope that this book will help bridge some of the inequalities and that a more comprehensive cancer center will lead to better outcomes for cancer patients. The information provided by the book shall serve as a backbone to assist centers obtain necessary resources to provide the best possible cancer care. We are pleased to be able to offer this book to the community and look forward to developing more best practices as we go forward in tackling these diseases.

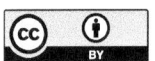

Chapter 2
Building a Comprehensive Cancer Center: Overall Structure

Dolores Grosso, Mahmoud Aljurf, and Usama Gergis

Introduction

According to the World Health Organization (WHO), cancer is the second leading cause of death globally, accounting for approximately 9.6 million deaths [1]. The WHO recommends that each nation has a national cancer control program (NCCP) to reduce the incidence of cancer and deaths related to cancer, as well as to improve the quality of life of cancer patients [2]. Comprehensive cancer centers form the backbone of a NCCP and are charged with developing innovative approaches to cancer prevention, diagnosis, and treatment [3]. This is accomplished through basic and clinical research, the provision of patient care, the training of new clinicians and scientists, and community outreach and education. Most comprehensive cancer centers are affiliated with university medical centers, but their cancer care initiatives may involve partnering outside the institution with other comprehensive cancer centers, community leaders, or members of industry [3]. When affiliated with a university medical center, cancer center executives must work in concert with their counterparts at the hospital, patient practice, medical school, and allied health science leaders resulting in an overlapping, often complicated reporting structure. Comprehensive cancer centers and the departments in the center receive funding for their services from various sources, including national and local grants, institutional funds, private donations, and industry [4].

The structure of a comprehensive cancer center arises from the mission of the center and the framework required to support this mission. The overarching

D. Grosso (✉) · U. Gergis
Medical Oncology, Thomas Jefferson University Hospital, Philadelphia, PA, USA
e-mail: dolores.grosso@jefferson.edu

M. Aljurf
Adult Hematology and HSCT, Oncology Centre, King Faisal Specialist Hospital & Research Centre, Riyadh, Saudi Arabia

© The Author(s) 2022
M. Aljurf et al. (eds.), *The Comprehensive Cancer Center*,
https://doi.org/10.1007/978-3-030-82052-7_2

3

mission of a comprehensive cancer center is to reduce the incidence of cancer and increase the quality of life and survival rates in patients with malignancies. There are three primary areas of cancer care: research, clinical care, and education that coalesce to meet this goal. Multiple interconnected departments are required to meet the objectives of the cancer center. Department heads include physicians, scientists, or administrators, depending on the focus of the department. The department leaders report to the comprehensive cancer center director, who is assisted by deputy directors and hospital advisory boards. The comprehensive cancer center director is typically an accomplished individual trained in a specific area of cancer research, but who has a vision for the broad research and clinical base required of the cancer center. The cancer center director has a multitude of responsibilities, including setting departmental goals, coordinating efforts between departments, hiring and retaining scientific staff, obtaining national, state, and philanthropic funding, creating new programs, and monitoring the business aspects of the center.

Structure of a Comprehensive Cancer Center Based on Mission

Research

Basic Laboratory Research

Basic laboratory research generates the knowledge that forms the basis for applied science. This type of research focuses on the mechanistic understanding of biochemical, biologic, physiologic, and pharmacologic processes as they relate to cancer and cancer treatments [5]. Tools used in this type of research include laboratory techniques such as flow cytometry analysis, bioimaging, spectroscopy, and gene sequencing. Laboratory experiments with human cell lines or animal models may also be utilized in this type of research. Basic laboratory research requires trained scientists, laboratory space and equipment, storage facilities for cell samples and cell lines, and areas for the humane care and housing of research animals. In most comprehensive cancer centers, a centralized source of core services and equipment exists, which is accessible to all scientists. Gene expression analysis and next-generation sequencing are examples of services provided by a comprehensive cancer center's core laboratory facility. Training of future generations of scientists is also a key function of laboratory scientists. Students in MD/PhD programs, clinical fellows requiring research experience, and postdoctoral scientists are examples of the many individuals trained in basic science in comprehensive cancer centers. The basic science division is composed of subspecialty areas such as immunology, cancer biology, or microbiology. Directors of these areas report to a director of basic science who in turn reports to the comprehensive cancer center director or deputy director.

Clinical Research in Human Subjects

Patients with cancer require multidisciplinary care to achieve optimal outcomes. Therefore, clinicians with expertise in medical, surgical, and radiation oncology participate in the direct care of patients with oncologic diagnoses and perform research in their specialty areas with the goal of improving cancer care. Examples of clinical research initiatives include those testing cancer prevention strategies [6], analyses of medication efficacy, trials comparing the benefits of various treatment modalities, and analyses of risk based on tumor genetic signature. Cancer research trials may be observational, analyzing cause and effect relationships, or interventional with the goal of evaluating the impact of a specific treatment [7]. Investigators in comprehensive cancer centers may participate with other institutions in national or international networks to analyze the outcomes of large numbers of combined patients providing more power to detect meaningful trends. Clinical research involves human subjects and, therefore, this type of research approach requires systems to be in place within the comprehensive cancer center to protect the safety, welfare, and rights of human research subjects.

Translational Research

Translational research is the integration of basic laboratory research with patient- and population-based research [8]. In this area, clinical research and basic research are complementary to each other with both areas contributing to a specific outcome. Ideally, translational research applies newly developed basic research understandings and applies them to early phase clinical research. This is a multistep, bidirectional process in which optimal treatments are refined over time by incremental discovery in both the clinical and laboratory settings. The ability to translate scientific data generated by the cancer center into actionable improvement in cancer care is central to the mission of the comprehensive cancer center. Therefore, a specific department of translational research exists in most cancer centers. Initiatives that foster working relationships between bench scientists and clinicians, such as scientific meetings, data sharing sessions, and availability of funding for multidisciplinary research, assist in the development of transitional research. Clinical trials, such as first-in-man or phase I studies, are developed by basic scientists and clinicians and are conducted within the comprehensive cancer center. The director of translational research reports directly to the comprehensive cancer center director or deputy director.

Population Health Research

The goal of population health science is to optimize health outcomes in specific populations. This type of research assesses trends in cancer incidence, identifies disparities in health care and suggests corrective actions, and examines cancer prevention, incidence, and treatment based on gender, race, or ethnicity, geographic location, or income. In doing so, population health scientists study community characteristics to inform the development of cancer care initiatives. In many comprehensive cancer centers, community outreach via education programs and free health services are offered through the population health department. The Framingham study is an early, important example of population health science which linked cigarette smoking, poor diet, and lack of exercise to the development of cardiovascular disease [9]. A more recent analysis of prostate cancer screening recommended different screening guidelines for African American versus Caucasian men, as African American men have a higher incidence and rate of death of prostate cancer than their Caucasian counterparts [10]. Population health scientists are in key positions to examine local health issues and can have direct, positive impacts on the health of their communities. The director of population health reports directly to the cancer center director or deputy director.

Protection of Human Subjects

Institutional Review Boards

The primary group responsible for the oversight of clinical research in human subjects is the Institutional Review Board (IRB) that reviews, approves, and monitors the conduct of clinical trials. Physicians, nurses, pharmacists, administrators, and community members can all serve on an IRB. The IRB reviews informed consent documents, investigator brochures, and provides guidance to investigators. The IRB also serves a critical role in monitoring the compliance of researchers to the conditions set forth in their clinical trials as well as adherence to IRB regulations for patient safety, sponsor-investigator relationships, reporting of adverse events, and adherence to national guidelines. IRBs follow guidelines set forth by national regulatory institutions. In the United States, IRBs follow good clinical practice and clinical trial guidelines set forth by the Food and Drug Administration and assure that researchers are trained in the basic principles of human research [11]. Most IRBs are part of the academic medical center that is affiliated with the comprehensive cancer center, but commercial and free-standing IRBs exist as well.

Clinical Research Organizations

Comprehensive cancer centers may utilize either in-house or contracted organizations to assist in the conduct of clinical trials. These clinical research organizations (CROs) assist the investigator in maintaining good clinical practices in the conduct of the clinical trial [12]. A CRO can provide a diverse array of services that include clinical and regulatory support of clinical trials. Examples of clinical services include procurement and shipping of clinical samples and supplies, development of case report forms, data capture of trial outcomes, adverse event monitoring, recording and reporting, trial pre-screening, and assistance with patient education and consent. Regulatory support includes developing standard operating procedures for compliance monitoring, audits to assess for compliance to trial procedures, and support for changing and updating clinical trial documents. Regulatory staff additionally facilitate communication between the sponsors and investigators of clinical trials and assist with the registration of clinical trials and clinical trial results to public and national databases. The department head managing an in-house CRO or who contracts with hired CROs reports to the comprehensive cancer center director or deputy director.

Other Key Programs Supporting Cancer Research

The goal of comprehensive cancer centers is to apply resources to projects that are scientifically rigorous, are likely to advance cancer prevention, care, and quality of life, and have the potential for benefitting the largest amount of people. Towards that end, committees that evaluate the scientific merit, the financial feasibility, and the appropriateness of proposed research projects to the identified research needs of the population are required. Other supportive programs include an Office of Biostatistics to assist in formulating research plans as well as analyzing trial outcomes. An office of technology transfer is important in the identification of novel ideas, assistance with the development and application of these ideas, as well as protection of intellectual rights.

Clinical Care of Patients with Cancer

The complexity of cancer diagnostics, treatment, and follow-up requires care across multiple disciplines [13]. Surgeons, interventional radiologists, and clinical practitioners are utilized to obtain tissue for pathological analysis. Accurate cancer diagnosis and prognostication depends upon the availability of pathologists trained in the analysis of cancer cells and accompanying genetic and molecular profiling. Radiology services are required for cancer staging and surveillance. Clinicians experienced in the treatment and administration of chemotherapy, oncology-based pharmacists, radiation oncologists, and surgeons specializing in oncology are required for the administration of treatment and the monitoring of response. The framework for this treatment includes inpatient and outpatient treatment areas, support staff, insurance, budgetary and billing staff, housekeeping, supply chain management resources, and equipment. In free-standing comprehensive cancer centers, directors of these areas report to the cancer center director. However, in comprehensive cancer centers affiliated with university medical centers, services are shared across all disciplines, although oncology-dedicated subdivisions within these departments exist. Cancer-specific specialty services within various specialties, such as cardiology, renal, and pulmonary, have been developed for more optimal management of organ-specific toxicities related to cancer treatment. Clinicians providing cancer care in university medical center settings may have dual reporting relationships to both the comprehensive cancer center director and to hospital or university-based leadership.

Quality Monitoring in Cancer Care

Cancer care is a highly complex, high-risk, discipline characterized by rapid development of new therapies. To provide the safest and most effective care, comprehensive cancer centers must establish systems to assess and monitor the quality and safety of care. There are multiple components of a quality program, including the development of standardized processes to deliver care, monitoring adherence to established guidelines for care, assessment of compliance with established guidelines, and the development of procedures to improve care. Examples include the use of evidence-based clinical pathways when ordering chemotherapy [14], monitoring adherence to quality indicators, such as those developed by the Agency for Healthcare Research and Quality (AHRQ), and medical record auditing to monitor compliance to national best practice standards, such as those set forth by the Foundation for the Accreditation of Cellular Therapy (FACT) [15], in stem cell transplant programs. Because quality initiatives are integrated into every department in the cancer center, there is typically an executive level position in the cancer center overseeing all aspects of the quality program. This executive reports directly to the cancer center director or deputy director.

Improving the Quality of Life of Cancer Patients: Support Services

Social Work

Social work is a mandatory discipline in every comprehensive cancer center supporting every aspect of a patient's cancer care experience. Social workers provide a wide array of patient services, including patient and family counseling and recognition of distress [16], assistance in finding financial reimbursement for medications and housing, end-of-life counseling and assistance with end-of-life issues [17]. Social workers have a broad array of responsibilities that may range from assistance in obtaining wigs, development of education programs for patients and families, or even coordinating fundraising services for patients and their families in the community. From the standpoint of continuity of care, social workers provide key information regarding the ability to obtain medications and information regarding health insurance issues as the patients move from inpatient to outpatient settings. Social workers increase the quality of cancer care by serving as a nonclinical support system.

Palliative Care

Palliative care is another aspect of cancer care that has the goal of increasing the patient's quality of life. Palliative care specialists are physicians or advanced practice providers who address the needs of patients with life-threatening illnesses. The aim of palliative care providers is to manage symptoms and side effects of cancer care [18]. This may encompass direct interventions to treat pain, anxiety, or neuropathy related to cancer treatments. Palliative care specialists also address spiritual, social, and psychological issues with patients. In some cancer centers, oncology-specific psychiatrists are part of the palliative care team. The palliative care team, in conjunction with clinicians and social workers, also may serve as end-of-life counselors. Palliative care specialists work in a variety of settings and are often available for acute issues in the inpatient and outpatient settings.

Navigation

Patients undergoing cancer care attempt to negotiate the complex health care system at a time of physical and psychological stress. Many cancer centers employ navigators to guide patients through the healthcare continuum. Navigators provide direct assistance to patients in making appointments, transferring records between offices, distributing directions to testing sites, coordinating family meetings, and providing a consistent contact for patients throughout cancer treatment. Navigators are also useful in providing consumer feedback to the cancer center to help improve services. Navigators have been shown to increase satisfaction and survival [19]. Most comprehensive cancer centers have some type of navigator services to support consistency and quality of care of patients with cancer. Registered nurses or specially trained lay people may serve as navigators in the comprehensive cancer center.

Survivorship

Survivorship refers to the physical, psychological, psychosocial, economic, and spiritual well-being of patients who have survived a cancer diagnosis [20]. Posttreatment survivorship goals include the transition back to a primary care provider for the majority of medical care, reintegration into the workforce, and return to family and social functions. This period of time in patient recovery may be marked by considerable anxiety related to both internal and external forces. Individuals recovered from cancer therapy have physical and mental challenges such as limited activity due to neuropathy, deconditioning, or osteoporosis, decreased self-confidence, or even fear of infection or relapse. Work supervisors may have concerns regarding the ability of returning employees to be fully productive. Family members, friends, and coworkers may have altered perceptions of cancer survivors resulting in relationship strain. Time missed from school or employment delays scholastic or career progression adding to frustration, stress, and anxiety. Comprehensive cancer centers support lifestyle reintegration through direct counseling and education from the clinical team, educational classes in the community sponsored by social workers, and the sponsorship of initiatives such as the buddy program, cancer survivor scholarships, beauty and support days, and job counselling.

Education

Comprehensive cancer centers are not only central to the education of future scientists and health care providers, but also take part in the development and continuing education of employees, patients, and the public via community outreach programs. When affiliated with a university medical center, cancer centers participate in the education of medical students, house staff, laboratory-based future scientists, and students from across all health science disciplines. Care of patients with cancer and cancer research is intertwined with academic faculty support and career progression resulting in ongoing research in cancer specialty areas. Grand rounds programs with internal or external speakers educate staff and students to new scientific discovery. Cancer centers also form partnerships with community leaders, government agencies, and industry to develop community outreach programs to improve health literacy, develop early detection programs, and raise money for cancer research.

Comprehensive cancer centers are highly complex institutions responsible for the advancement of cancer research, clinical care, and education. A multitude of personnel with varying areas of expertise are responsible for the integration of all the critical cancer center activities described in this chapter. Therefore, a highly organized and functional framework is necessary to avoid overlap and address all aspects of the cancer center's mission. Figure 2.1 displays the basic organization chart of a university-affiliated comprehensive cancer center.

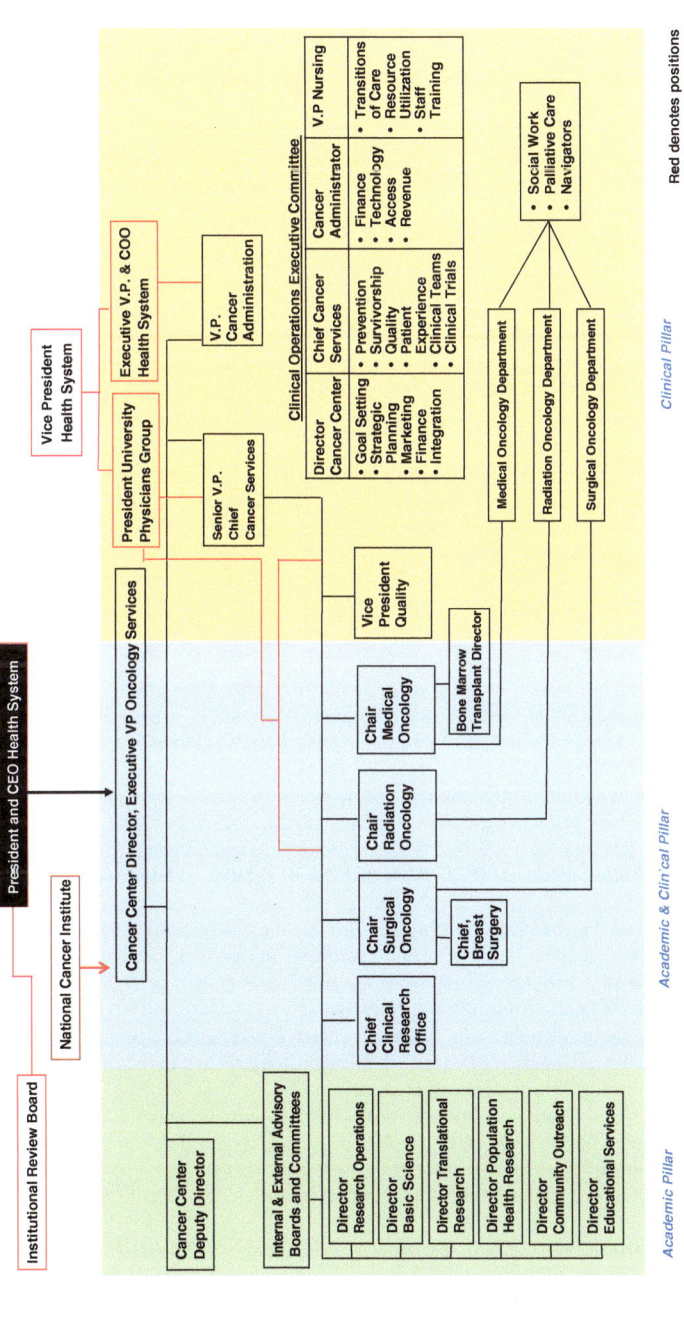

Fig. 2.1 Structure of a comprehensive cancer center that is affiliated with a university medical center. In this example, the mission of the comprehensive cancer center is divided into three pillars. Personnel in the Academic Pillar provide academic leadership and planning of cancer center goals. The Academic and Clinical Pillar is composed of clinician leaders who assure that the goals of the cancer center are brought to individual departments, while the Clinical Pillar is composed primarily of clinicians and other key individuals providing direct patient care. Individuals in all three pillars ultimately report to the comprehensive cancer center director

References

1. World Health Organization. Cancer. 2020. Accessed May 6, 2020 at: https://www.who.int/health-topics/cancer#tab=tab_1.
2. World Health Organization. National cancer care programmes. 2020. Accessed May 6, 2020 at: https://www.who.int/cancer/nccp/en/.
3. National Cancer Institute. NCI-designated cancer centers. 2018. Accessed May 6, 2020 at: https://www.cancer.gov/research/nci-role/cancer-centers.
4. Eckhouse S, Sullivan R. A survey of public funding of cancer research in the European union. PLoS Med. 2006;3(7):e267.
5. Association of American Medical Colleges-AAMC. Basic science. 2020. Accessed May 6, 2020 at: https://www.aamc.org/what-we-do/mission-areas/medical-research/basic-science.
6. McCaskill-Stevens W, Pearson DC, Kramer BS, Ford LG, Lippman SM. Identifying and creating the next generation of community-based cancer prevention studies: summary of a National Cancer Institute think tank. Cancer Prev Res (Phila). 2017;10(2):99–107.
7. Thiese MS. Observational and interventional study design types; an overview. Biochem Med. 2014;24(2):199–210.
8. Rubio DM, Schoenbaum EE, Lee LS, et al. Defining translational research: implications for training. Acad Med. 2010;85(3):470–5.
9. Mahmood S, Levy D, Vasan R, Wang T. The Framingham Heart Study and the epidemiology of cardiovascular disease: a historical perspective. Lancet. 2014;383(9921):P999–1008.
10. Shenoy D, Packianathan S, Chen AM, Vijayakumar S. Do African-American men need separate prostate cancer screening guidelines? BMC Urol. 2016;16(1):19.
11. U.S. Food and Drug Administration. Institutional review boards (IRBs) protection of human subjects in clinical trials. Sept 11, 2019. Accessed May 8, 2020 at: https://www.fda.gov/about-fda/center-drug-evaluation-and-research-cder/institutional-review-boards-irbs-and-protection-human-subjects-clinical-trials.
12. World Health Organization. Handbook for good research clinical practice. 2002. Accessed May 11, 2020 at: https://www.who.int/medicines/areas/quality_safety/safety_efficacy/gcp1.pdf.
13. Taylor C, Munro AJ, Glynne-Jones R, et al. Multidisciplinary team working in cancer: what is the evidence? BMJ. 2010;340:c951.
14. Ellis PG. Development and implementation of oncology care pathways in an integrated care network: the via oncology pathways experience. J Oncol Pract. 2013;9(3):171–3.
15. Foundation for the Accreditation of Cellular Therapy. Setting the global standard for top quality patient care in cellular therapies. 2020. Accessed May 12, 2020 at: http://www.factwebsite.org/.
16. Pirl WF, Fann JR, Greer JA, et al. Recommendations for the implementation of distress screening programs in cancer centers: report from the American Psychosocial Oncology Society (APOS), Association of Oncology Social Work (AOSW), and Oncology Nursing Society (ONS) joint task force. Cancer. 2014;120(19):2946–54.
17. Becker F. Oncology social workers' role in patient-centered care. 2017. Accessed May 15, 2020 at: https://www.accc-cancer.org/acccbuzz/blog-post-template/accc-buzz/2017/03/15/oncology-social-workers-role-in-patient-centered-care.
18. National Institute of Health: National Cancer Institute. Palliative care in cancer. 2017. Accessed May 15, 2020 at: https://www.cancer.gov/about-cancer/advanced-cancer/care-choices/palliative-care-fact-sheet.
19. Riley S, Riley C. The role of patient navigation in improving the value of oncology care. J Clin Pathw. 2016;2(1):41–7.
20. McCanney J, Winckworth-Prejsnar K, Schatz A, et al. Addressing survivorship in cancer care. J Natl Compr Cancer Netw. 2018;16(7):802–7.

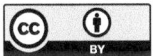

Chapter 3
The Inpatient Unit in a Cancer Center

Mohamed A. Kharfan-Dabaja

Introduction

Treatment of cancer has evolved significantly over the past four decades, moving away from traditional chemotherapies, with or without radiation therapy, to smarter targeted therapies [1–3]. As many of these novel treatments became available in oral formulations, or as short intravenous infusions or through the subcutaneous route, this has allowed moving several regimens to be administered in the outpatient setting. This is the case for a significant number of cancer treatment regimens for diseases, such as chronic lymphocytic (CLL) and chronic myelogenous (CML) leukemias, for which the current standard therapies are administered orally [4, 5]; and for various solid neoplasms, namely, lung, breast, colon, and prostate cancer, among others, for which contemporary regimens lend themselves for administration in outpatient infusion centers. The increase in health care cost has also played an important role on supporting shifting cancer care to the outpatient setting [6].

Yet, a significant number of patients still require treatment in the inpatient setting, owing to the nature of the treatment, duration, and frequency, or to the level of supportive care required to administer such treatments, among others. Presently, the majority of cases treated in the inpatient setting include induction and consolidation therapies for acute leukemias, myeloid (AML) or lymphoid (ALL), and certain biotherapies [7, 8]. This also applies to more complex procedures like hematopoietic cell transplantation (HCT), particularly allogeneic HCT (allo-HCT), and chimeric antigen receptor T-cell therapy (CAR T) [9–13]. In the case of autologous HCT (auto-HCT), some regimens used for lymphomas are preferentially prescribed for administration in the inpatient setting, while using high-dose melphalan for

M. A. Kharfan-Dabaja (✉)
Division of Hematology-Oncology, Mayo Clinic, Jacksonville, FL, USA

Blood and Marrow Transplantation Program, Mayo Clinic, Jacksonville, FL, USA
e-mail: KharfanDabaja.Mohamed@mayo.edu

© The Author(s) 2022
M. Aljurf et al. (eds.), *The Comprehensive Cancer Center*,
https://doi.org/10.1007/978-3-030-82052-7_3

15

multiple myeloma is commonly offered in the outpatient setting. Furthermore, some cancer patients may need to be hospitalized for management of their symptoms, such as intractable pain or treatment of infection(s) requiring frequent antimicrobial dosing, or for nutritional support; and/or many other complications that might have resulted from cancer treatment. In many inpatient units at cancer centers, private rooms are also available for patients who need palliative or hospice care.

Apart from specialized trained physicians and nurses, the number of inpatient team services has expanded significantly to meet the complex needs of patients and their families. Pharmacists are resourceful to help understand, guide, and manage the potential side effects of new therapies and to educate patients to better understand cancer treatment and potential benefits and complications. The pharmacy team, in coordination with physicians, nurses, and clinical research coordinators, also plays a crucial role in safeguarding the well-being of patients who are participating in clinical trials evaluating safety and efficacy of new drugs. Oncology social workers and case managers have also become an integral part of inpatient teams helping provide psychosocial support, and assist with short- or long- term placement, whenever warranted, and to coordinate discharge needs by planning and identifying needed resources for a smooth transition to the outpatient setting. Certified nutritionists, dieticians, and physical and occupational therapists are also available to assist with clinical interventions. During cancer treatment, it is also important to recognize the importance of addressing the patients' spiritual needs.

There is not a universal model for how an inpatient unit should be built and developed. This would certainly depend on several aspects including financial resources, population density, and societal factors, among others. Below, we attempt to describe the main components of an inpatient cancer treatment unit. We divide them into the human factor and other factors.

The Human Factor

Successful operation of an inpatient unit is certainly dependent on a complex and well-orchestrated multidisciplinary approach to cancer care. The inpatient unit also provides an opportunity to educate future generation of physicians, advanced practice providers, and nurses in various specialties and subspecialties, particularly hematology, medical and surgical oncology, infectious diseases, and psychiatry, among others.

The model most commonly applied in teaching hospitals comprises an inpatient attending physician that is responsible for leading and coordinating the care of patients. The team also includes trainees, generally hematology and/or medical oncology fellows and internal medicine residents, medical students, advanced practice providers, namely, physician assistants and advanced registered nurse practitioners, nurses, a pharmacist, a social worker, and a case manager. Nutritionists and physical and occupational therapists are also called upon to participate in patient care based on indicated needs. In more complex procedures like hematopoietic cell transplantation, there is ample participation of subspecialties such as infectious diseases owing to the increased risks of opportunistic infections in the setting of profound immune suppression. For patients receiving CAR T-cell therapy, there is active participation from specialties such as neuro-oncology owing to potential-associated neurotoxicity and intensive care unit specialists. Other specialties may also end up participating in the care of CAR T-cell recipients if they develop organ failure; for example, nephrologists in the case of renal failure and cardiology in the case of cardiac dysfunction, among others. In the nonacademic community setting, similar multidisciplinary services are also available; and some community-based cancer centers also provide educational and training opportunities.

Nurses play an important role in the inpatient oncology setting as they are directly involved in the care of patients and generally the first to become aware of any change in a patient's clinical condition [14]. Patients' perceptions of excellence in healthcare are strongly associated with nursing care [15]. There is not an established standard pertaining to a nurse-to-patient ratio in an oncology inpatient unit; and staffing needs depends on various factors including, but not limited to, level of acuity, volume of patients in the unit, and nursing skills in the case of complex procedures such as allo-HCT or CAR T-cell therapy. Thorough assessment of these patients is crucial to ensure optimal care and timely intervention whenever needed. For instance, oral mucositis and gastrointestinal toxicities are commonly seen when patients are prescribed high doses of chemotherapy as it could be the case of certain induction regimens for AML or ALL; or conditioning regimens for autologous HCT (auto-HCT) or allo-HCT which may also involve radiotherapy, resulting in serious malnutrition. Nurses would generally be the first to become aware of such findings and alert the rest of the team to consult nutritionists to help incorporate enteral or parenteral strategies to optimize patient's nutritional status. Several studies have reported adverse outcomes and nurse burnout with higher patients-to-nurse ratios [16, 17]. A recently published meta-analytical study showed considerable risk of burnout, emotional exhaustion, and depersonalization in nursing professionals in oncology services [18].

Other Factors

Floor Design

Inpatient cancer units are designed to provide the safest and most efficient care for patients. Generally, the floor layout is designed to position nurses in close proximity to the patients' beds to be able to respond more promptly to patient's needs. A work station is located right outside the door or inside the room (Fig. 3.1). This design is meant to improve efficiency and reduce the time spent away from patient care. In some facilities, central monitors are available to display important vital signs, such as monitoring of heart rate and blood pressure in patients who may be receiving certain types of chemotherapies, biological or experimental therapies. Yet, applicability of this design in underdeveloped countries may be challenging due to financial limitations or due to lack of technology.

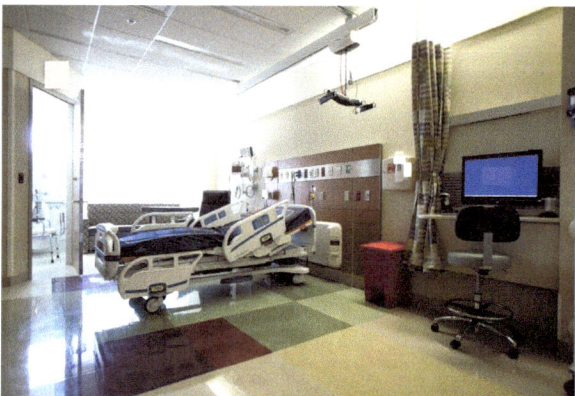

Fig. 3.1 Inpatient hospital room in a cancer floor, Mayo Clinic, Jacksonville, FL, USA. (Used with permission of Mayo Foundation for Medical Education and Research, all rights reserved)

Environmental

The complex inpatient cancer center environment demands special consideration to ensure a healthy indoor air quality to protect patients against hospital-acquired infections [19, 20]. Sources of air pollution within the hospital include chemicals and microbial air pollutants from various sources [21]. Properly designed systems and optimal operations are essential to control and mitigate potential sources of pollutants such as air filtration, differential pressure control, directional airflow control, and ultraviolet germicidal irradiation disinfection, among others [22].

Rooms

The majority of cancer centers in the United States would provide a private room to a cancer patient in need of inpatient care. Naturally, a private room would offer a more restful and healing environment. Nevertheless, a private room is a necessity for those patients who require contact or respiratory isolation. In the case of patients undergoing a HCT or CAR-T therapy, these procedures are better administered in the setting of a private hospital room owing to the high risk of serious infections in the setting of profound cytopenias and immune suppression. With the advent of electronic health records, nowadays rooms are equipped with a work station inside the room (Fig. 3.1) for both convenience and efficacy.

Positive Pressure Rooms

Positively pressurized rooms are generally considered the cleanest environments in a hospital. A room is pressurized so that it is positive with respect to adjacent areas. It is designed in such a way to protect severely immunocompromised patients from possible airborne pathogens present in adjacent areas. Positively pressurized rooms also commonly use high-efficiency particulate air (HEPA) filters at the supply terminals to guarantee the highest air quality to the patient. These types of rooms are generally found in Blood and Marrow Transplant units.

Negative Pressure Rooms

Conversely, negatively pressurized rooms used for airborne infection isolation are engineered to prevent airborne microbial contaminants from flowing to other areas. These rooms are generally reserved for patients who develop infections like tuberculosis because the organism can spread in the air from the patient to members of the healthcare team. The room typically is served by a dedicated exhaust fan, and some facilities also use UV radiation for disinfecting purposes.

Discussion

We described the main components of an inpatient unit in a cancer center. The ultimate goal must be to provide a safe environment for cancer patients and to facilitate delivery of care in an efficient manner. As healthcare expenditure continues to rise, it is important to ensure long-term sustainability by minimizing as much as possible operating costs.

Despite all advances, there are continuous challenges pertaining to further improving safety in the inpatient cancer setting. These include, but are not limited to, prevention of falls, nosocomial infections, and medication errors. Establishing interdisciplinary working groups which involve all healthcare participants and incorporate new technologies would certainly prove essential to further improve the safety and quality of care for patients with cancer.

Conflicts of Interests The author discloses consultancy for Pharmacyclics and Daiichi Sankyo.

References

1. Topper MJ, et al. The emerging role of epigenetic therapeutics in immuno-oncology. Nat Rev Clin Oncol. 2020;17(2):75–90.
2. Paz-Ares L, et al. Pembrolizumab plus chemotherapy for squamous non-small-cell lung cancer. N Engl J Med. 2018;379(21):2040–51.
3. Schmid P, et al. Pembrolizumab for early triple-negative breast cancer. N Engl J Med. 2020;382(9):810–21.
4. Woyach JA, et al. Ibrutinib regimens versus chemoimmunotherapy in older patients with untreated CLL. N Engl J Med. 2018;379(26):2517–28.
5. Kantarjian H, et al. Dasatinib versus imatinib in newly diagnosed chronic-phase chronic myeloid leukemia. N Engl J Med. 2010;362(24):2260–70.

6. Mariotto AB, et al. Projections of the cost of cancer care in the United States: 2010-2020. J Natl Cancer Inst. 2011;103(2):117–28.
7. Lancet JE, et al. CPX-351 (cytarabine and daunorubicin) liposome for injection versus conventional cytarabine plus daunorubicin in older patients with newly diagnosed secondary acute myeloid leukemia. J Clin Oncol. 2018;36(26):2684–92.
8. Kantarjian H, et al. Blinatumomab versus chemotherapy for advanced acute lymphoblastic leukemia. N Engl J Med. 2017;376(9):836–47.
9. Kharfan-Dabaja MA, et al. Haematopoietic cell transplantation for blastic plasmacytoid dendritic cell neoplasm: a North American multicentre collaborative study. Br J Haematol. 2017;179(5):781–9.
10. Kharfan-Dabaja MA, et al. Allogeneic hematopoietic cell transplantation for Richter syndrome: a single-center experience. Clin Lymphoma Myeloma Leuk. 2018;18(1):e35–9.
11. Kharfan-Dabaja MA, et al. Higher busulfan dose intensity appears to improve leukemia-free and overall survival in AML allografted in CR2: an analysis from the Acute Leukemia Working Party of the European Group for Blood and Marrow Transplantation. Leuk Res. 2015;39(9):933–7.
12. Neelapu SS, et al. Axicabtagene ciloleucel CAR T-cell therapy in refractory large B-cell lymphoma. N Engl J Med. 2017;377(26):2531–44.
13. Schuster SJ, et al. Tisagenlecleucel in adult relapsed or refractory diffuse large B-cell lymphoma. N Engl J Med. 2019;380(1):45–56.
14. Musy SN, et al. Longitudinal study of the variation in patient turnover and patient-to-nurse ratio: descriptive analysis of a Swiss University Hospital. J Med Internet Res. 2020;22(4):e15554.
15. Aiken LH, et al. Patient satisfaction with hospital care and nurses in England: an observational study. BMJ Open. 2018;8(1):e019189.
16. Cho SH, et al. Nurse staffing, nurses prioritization, missed care, quality of nursing care, and nurse outcomes. Int J Nurs Pract. 2020;26(1):e12803.
17. Wang QQ, et al. Job burnout and quality of working life among Chinese nurses: a cross-sectional study. J Nurs Manag. 2019;27(8):1835–44.
18. Canadas-De la Fuente GA, et al. Prevalence of burnout syndrome in oncology nursing: a meta-analytic study. Psychooncology. 2018;27(5):1426–33.
19. Leung M, Chan AH. Control and management of hospital indoor air quality. Med Sci Monit. 2006;12(3):SR17–23.
20. El-Sharkawy MF, Noweir ME. Indoor air quality levels in a University Hospital in the Eastern Province of Saudi Arabia. J Family Community Med. 2014;21(1):39–47.
21. McLarnon NA, et al. The efficiency of an air filtration system in the hospital ward. Int J Environ Health Res. 2006;16(4):313–7.
22. Benet T, et al. Reduction of invasive aspergillosis incidence among immunocompromised patients after control of environmental exposure. Clin Infect Dis. 2007;45(6):682–6.

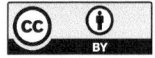

Chapter 4
Outpatient Care

Ian Qianhuang Wu, Francesca Lorraine Wei Inng Lim, and Liang Piu Koh

Haematology and oncology departments have historically required inpatient ward beds for a large number of their treatments. There are many reasons for this, including the administration of complex and lengthy intravenous regimens and significant treatment-related toxicities such as emetogenicity, mucositis and infections. Over the last 20 years, however, there has been a move for selected patients to be managed in the outpatient setting, for both chemotherapy regimens and hematopoietic stem cell transplants (HSCTs). This has been done both during treatment and in the monitoring period following immediately afterwards. The outpatient environment ranges from the oncology office, outpatient hospital department, accommodation-based treatment facilities including hotels, to even the patients' own homes.

This change has mostly been driven by several factors:

1. Increasing pressure on the capacity of inpatient facilities and rationalization of inpatient beds
2. Avoidance of unnecessary hospitalization
3. Improvement in cost-efficiency
4. Improvement of patient experience [1]

Several other additional factors have aided in the transition of cancer care to the outpatient setting. The availability of mobile infusion devices for chemotherapy, good supportive care and medications, as well as the development of targeted cancer therapies are just a few. In the United States, the push towards outpatient care was also aided by non-medical factors such as regulatory and economic ones – the

I. Q. Wu · L. P. Koh (✉)
Department of Hematology-Oncology, National University Cancer Institute, National University Health System, Singapore, Singapore
e-mail: liang_piu_koh@nuhs.edu.sg

F. L. W. I. Lim
Department of Hematology, Singapore General Hospital, SingHealth, Singapore, Singapore

M. Aljurf et al. (eds.), *The Comprehensive Cancer Center*,
https://doi.org/10.1007/978-3-030-82052-7_4

Medicare Prescription Drug Improvement and Modernization Act of 2003 changing the calculus of infusion therapy reimbursements.

Outpatient care in haematology-oncology centres provide many benefits, including:

1. Reducing the inpatient clinical load and alleviating pressure on constrained healthcare resources in order to optimize care delivery to high-acuity patients.
2. Giving patients freedom from the hospital environment, providing families time together and allowing a degree of normality to remain. The ability to stay out of a hospital setting in a smaller, more comforting and familiar environment is often linked with higher patient satisfaction [2]. In addition, it also allows patients and caregivers to take back some control and become active members of the treatment team.
3. Survivorship programs – transitioning to primary care providers so oncologists can spend more time with newly diagnosed patients
4. Cost-effectiveness: Ambulatory care is recognized as a cost-saving initiative. Savings can be found in bed days [3] and staffing expenditure. A study at University College London Hospital [1] estimated that nurse staffing for their ambulatory care service cost approximately a third of that of the inpatient equivalent. It is important to emphasize that the amount of cost efficacy is heavily dependent on local regulations and reimbursement policies.

A multidisciplinary approach is crucial to the successful delivery of outpatient haematology and oncology care. A team of clinicians, pharmacists and nurses are just a few of many different disciplines crucial to the smooth running of an outpatient service. Ancillary services can also be offered in an outpatient setting, including nutrition and dietetics, physical therapy, psychological care as well as transitory services. Efforts should be made at planning level to coordinate seamless care in the ambulatory setting, focusing on synergy, access, synchronization and patient satisfaction.

Clinicians

Clinicians are crucial in identifying patients that may be appropriate for outpatient cancer care, as well as leveraging on their therapeutic relationship with the patient to encourage and educate them [4]. The primary oncologist plays a key role in coordinating and utilizing the various services that are available at each unique center.

Cancer is a complex condition that requires close cooperation with not just the primary oncologist, but several other disciplines as well. These typically include surgical specialties, radiation oncologists, infectious disease physicians and cardiologists. It is increasingly recognized that cancer patients have unique needs and disease profiles. With patients surviving longer and receiving increased numbers of lines of treatment, the types of complications experienced are also increasing. The role of multi-specialty clinics involving clinicians from various specialties is gaining in popularity as it can reduce the number of clinic visits a patient requires and also harmonizes care between the various disciplines.

Nursing and the Role of Advanced Practice Providers and Nurse Coordinators

It is impossible to overstate the role of nursing in an ambulatory cancer center. Oncology nurses are key to successful oncology care as they spend the most time with patients, playing the role of caregiver, educator, advocate and care coordinator. With the projected increase in oncology patient encounters expected to outpace that of anticipated resources, the ASCO Workforce Advisory Group has recommended improved integration of advanced practice providers (APPs) into the oncology workforce [5].

APPs can make significant contributions throughout a patient's journey with cancer – from detection and diagnosis, through treatment, survivorship, surveillance and even end-of-life care [6]. Training to become a Nurse Practitioner (NP) helps develop the individual's scientific foundation, leadership, quality improvement competencies, practice inquiry skills, technology and information literacy, policy competencies, health delivery system competencies, ethics competencies and independent practice competencies [7].

Besides the role of APPs, nurses also play an important role in their function as oncology nurse coordinators. As mentioned previously, cancer care is often complex and involves several moving parts that are centred around the patient. Key elements of a nurse coordinator's role involve emotional support, guidance to patients, and coordination of the multifaceted aspects of the patient's care [8].

Pharmacists, Drug Administration and Preparation

Pharmacists are essential to the running of any cancer center. Their role encompasses checking of prescriptions, drug preparation, and patient education. They play a major role in ensuring safe, effective and cost-effective drug therapy [9].

The availability of ambulatory delivery devices and hydration pumps is one of the key factors facilitating the move of so much inpatient clinical care to the ambulatory setting. These have enabled the ambulatory delivery of drugs such as ifosfamide and post-hydration for methotrexate regimens that were previously only administered on inpatient wards. The use of infusion pumps has enabled the ambulatory administration of regimens containing chemotherapy drugs typically given by continuous infusion (e.g. cisplatin in ESHAP) on an intermittent schedule (e.g. twice daily dosing), or those requiring continuous hydration fluid (e.g. ifosfamide or high-dose methotrexate-containing regimens). Several drugs previously administered intravenously were converted to oral administration to further facilitate outpatient administration. Specific examples include oral folinic acid and sodium bicarbonate for high-dose methotrexate regimens and oral mesna for oxazophosphorine-containing regimens, as well as antiemetics.

Optimal routes of outpatient drug administration need to be constantly evaluated to reduce chair times and ease of administration. Increasingly, several therapies are released in oral formulations, or may be able to be administered subcutaneously (e.g. CD20 monoclonal antibodies Rituximab for treatment of B cell lymphoma) rather than through prolonged intravenous infusions. This helps in optimizing chair usage and time spent for the patient.

Strategies that have been utilized to minimize wastage of chemotherapy drugs include

1. Prepacked medications
2. Dose banding
3. Same day chemotherapy

Many drugs either use a flat dose or have traditionally been based on calculations of the patient's body surface area (BSA). The use of BSA or other weight-based calculations for dosing of chemotherapy drugs have been controversial and may not be correlated with efficacy or toxicity. The advantages of dose banding and pre-packaging for more commonly used chemotherapy medications with longer drug stability can greatly reduce the time and manpower needed in the cancer center pharmacy to prepare them. A list of chemotherapy drugs that can be pre-packaged should be available in each outpatient pharmacy and referenced in the planning and organization of the centre's processes [10].

Supportive Care for Chemotherapy or HSCT-Related Complications

Delivery of good supportive care for haematology-oncology patients and stem cell transplant recipients is vital in ambulatory care. Nursing and medical staff running ambulatory care centres must be equipped with the knowledge and experience in the management of chemotherapy complication. Improved antiemetic regimens now allow patients to avoid nausea and vomiting that require admission for intravenous hydration and antiemetics. Outpatient monitoring following chemotherapy during the neutropenic phase has been shown to be safe for many regimens, including for highly intensive protocols such as consolidation chemotherapy for acute leukaemias. HSCTs have also been given in either a mixed inpatient–outpatient setting, or entirely outpatient. The largest series of autografts reported have been Melphalan autografts for myeloma [11] and BEAM (Carmustine, Etoposide, Cytarabine and Melphalan) autografts for lymphoma [12], although many others have performed

HSCT with reduced intensity conditioning or non-myeloablative regimens in outpatient settings as well [13].

Transfusion of blood products is also a common therapy that is administered in outpatient centres. An on-site blood transfusion service is most desirable for this purpose, although in the absence of one, this service can still be offered in collaboration with the blood transfusion service in closest proximity provided the appropriate safety and quality assurance measures are put in place.

Ancillary and Community Services

It is beneficial to an outpatient cancer center to provide ancillary services, although this will be dependent on the needs of the patient population each center serves. These services include physical therapy, nutrition and dietetics, and psychological services, amongst many others. A significant proportion of cancer patients can be malnourished and physically deconditioned from their illness [14], and can benefit greatly from having on-site services that address these needs. It is also estimated that about 32% of cancer patients are diagnosed with at least one mental disorder [15], supporting the need for psycho-oncology services.

In addition to on-site services, partnerships with local primary care providers and the setting up of satellite centres can also be explored. As an example, patients who require routine blood transfusions may be able to have this administered in a primary care or satellite center closer in proximity to their place of residence, rather than at the main cancer center. The same goes for procedures such as the flushing of lines, as well as blood tests. Medication delivery services could be explored for stable patients who do not require frequent physician reviews as this will also allow patients to maintain a normal life outside without spending too much time in a crowded clinic.

Planning for Outpatient Chemotherapy and Drug Delivery

Various models of delivering outpatient chemotherapy have been explored. The optimal model harmonizing physician appointments, blood tests, nursing services and chemotherapy administration needs to be unique to every center and the community it serves. For example, patients treated at a cancer center located in a busy urban community with well-connected infrastructure and transport will have different needs compared to those being treated in a regional center that may be more suitable for stable patients on maintenance therapies and do not require higher levels of nursing care.

The organization of an outpatient chemotherapy center does not only involve the administration of the chemotherapy drug, but also the process – involving

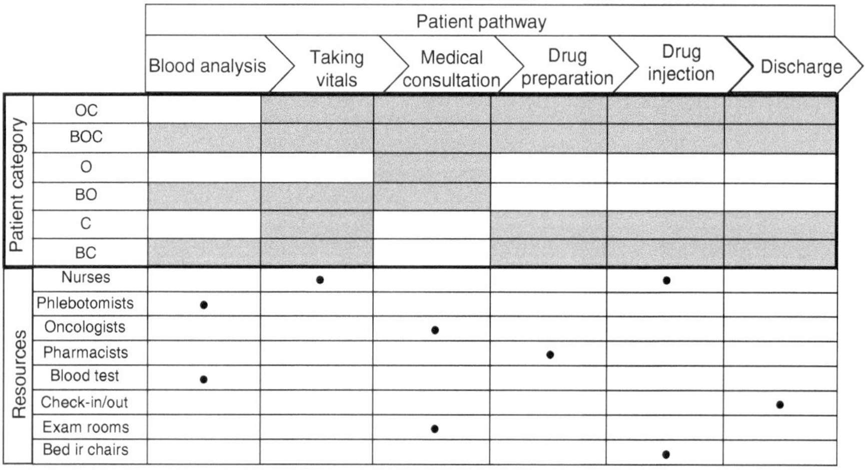

		Patient pathway					
		Blood analysis	Taking vitals	Medical consultation	Drug preparation	Drug injection	Discharge
Patient category	OC						
	BOC						
	O						
	BO						
	C						
	BC						
Resources	Nurses		•			•	
	Phlebotomists	•					
	Oncologists			•			
	Pharmacists				•		
	Blood test	•					
	Check-in/out						•
	Exam rooms			•			
	Bed ir chairs					•	

Fig. 4.1 Patient pathway for outpatient chemotherapy with patient categories and resources. (Lamé et al. [10])

consultations, blood tests and drug preparation, and the resources – both human and technical. An example of a patient pathway for a chemotherapy session is illustrated in Fig. 4.1. However, it is important to note that not every patient follows the same pathway – for example, some patients require blood tests prior to chemotherapy while some do not. Liang et al. (2015) [16] have described three categories: (i) OC – Oncologist appointment and Chemotherapy, (ii) O – Oncologist appointment only, (iii) C – Chemotherapy only. Further refinement has been suggested by Lame et al. (2016) [10] by the addition of a further distinction – whether the patient requires blood tests, B – resulting in six categories of OC, BOC, O, BO, C, BC. Resources then need to be allocated to these categories, including but not limited to, nurses, phlebotomists, pharmacists, examination rooms and chemotherapy suites.

The backbone of outpatient chemotherapy administration is largely similar across most centres, although variations in its organization are common and unique to each center. Lame et al. (2016) [10] has outlined options for organizational variants in outpatient chemotherapy pertaining to the chronological order various aspects of the chemotherapy process is performed (Table 4.1) [10]. Whichever model a center chooses to adopt, it is imperative that the focus remains on maximizing resources and minimizing wastage, while optimizing patient care and enhancing the patient experience.

For example, Lau et al. (2014) [17] showed that patients preferred chemotherapy on the same day as their oncology outpatient appointments. However, not all chemotherapy regimens can be administered as such due to factors such as drug preparation time, or duration of administration. Soh et al. (2015) [18] attempted to circumvent this through pre-packaging of chemotherapy to improve patient waiting times for chemotherapy. However, experience in the Netherlands Cancer Institute shows up to 10% of patients with blood tests, and 5% of those without, were

Table 4.1 Options for outpatient chemotherapy delivery

	Options	Advantages	Risks
Blood test	Chemo day in-house	Streamlined process	Patients wait
		Patients come only once	Sensitivity to equipment failures
	In-house on previous day	Reduced waiting time on chemo day	Patients must come two days in a row
	In external lab on previous day	Reduced waiting time on chemo day	Poor hospital-lab coordination leads to a lost advantage and is time consuming
		Freed hospital lab capacity for other (more urgent) analysis	
Drug preparation	Chemo day	Certainty on patient status: no wasted drugs	Patients wait
			Sensitivity to equipment failures
	Previous day	Drugs ready on patients' arrival if consultation is still on chemo day	Wasted drugs
	Mixt	Reduced waiting times	Patients with expensive drugs wait
		Less wasted drugs than 100% on previous day	Still some wasted drugs
Oncologist consultation	Chemo day	Patients come only once	No early confirmation on patient status: patients wait drug preparation
	Previous day	Less waiting time because drugs can be prepared in advance	Patients have to come two days in a row
		Possibility to start chemo earlier	
Nurse-patient allocation	Functional	Pooled resources: optimized utilization	Less possibility for patient-nurse connections
	Primary	Better patient-nurse connection	Lost productivity if the nurse's schedule cannot be filled

Lamé et al. [10]

eventually deemed unfit for treatment [19]. The potential for drug wastage and accompanying financial costs for such a strategy cannot be underestimated, further emphasizing the need to strike a fine balance between resource planning and patient experience.

It is important for centres to continuously collect data and regularly review organizational policies. Lean healthcare practices should be encouraged, and advances in technology should be evaluated to further this aim [20]. As an example, mathematical modelling can improve scheduling [16], and the use of technology like radio frequency identification (RFID) can optimize chair use and the number of patients served [21].

Economical Advantages of Outpatient Care

The financial benefits of running an outpatient cancer center is heavily dependent on local regulations and funding. The benefits and shortfalls will be heterogenous across many states and countries so local regulations need to be carefully examined and approached appropriately. If possible, cooperation with local public officials should be sought to make outpatient care an attractive option for all the other non-financial benefits outlined in this chapter.

Clinical Trials

Great advances have been made in haematology-oncology in the past few decades, and increased understanding of the immunology and biology of cancer has led to the development of many therapeutics. Clinical trials are important in assessing the safety and efficacy of any treatment and form a cornerstone of cancer care. Consideration should be given to the setting up of an outpatient clinical trial center that is geared for the running of phase 1 or phase 2 trials. These services can aid with the recruitment of patients and monitoring of parameters such as pharmacokinetic/pharmacodynamic studies. They can either form part of the outpatient clinic, or set up as an independent unit, depending on the size of the center.

Telemedicine

Telemedicine utilizes telecommunication technology to deliver healthcare services, including consults and education. It is also a tool that allows for multidisciplinary discussion, including telepathology. Communities that benefit the most from the utilization of telemedicine are those in areas physically distant from the center in which they normally receive care. Telemedicine has been tested in multiple areas of medicine (not limited to oncological care) and has demonstrated high levels of satisfaction in both patients and physicians [22]. Several studies have also demonstrated improved cost efficacy with telemedicine [23]. Telemedicine can be used to complement traditional methods of patient care, from expanding access to specialist support, to education and patient support [24].

It should be stressed that telemedicine is not just using mobile apps like FaceTime™ or Zoom™ to engage with a patient, even if patients may request for consults to be conducted in this manner for the sake of convenience. It is imperative that whichever telemedicine platform is utilized (whether a program developed in-house or a commercial one), due care is taken to protect patient and data confidentiality and security. Telemedicine services can be approached in two main ways – synchronous or asynchronous formats. The former involves real-time engagement between the patient and his physician utilizing interactive video technology. The latter involves a "store-forward" approach where clinical data elements such as imaging, lab results, and video recordings can be stored to be interpreted at a later time [22]. Measures need to be put in place for a successful telemedicine service in order to achieve patient outcomes and satisfaction that is at least equivalent to in-person consultation.

Apart from conducting consultations with patients, telemedicine can be utilized in other ways to augment the patient care experience, for both patients and healthcare providers alike. The increased development of wearables that can aid in remote monitoring of patients' vital signs may allow patients to be monitored at home for signs and symptoms of treatment-related complications such as fever [24]. Patient examination, with the exception of palpation, can also be performed with the right training and tools. Wound care, symptom management and even palliative care can also be administered using portable technology that can increase patient access to these services [22].

Telepathology is also an emerging technology that allows pathologists to remotely view microscopic images without being physically coupled to a microscope. The most discernible benefit thus far appears to be the accessibility to trained cytopathologists who are involved in rapid on-site evaluation (ROSE) of tissue obtained from minimally invasive procedures where the tissue sufficiency is integral to accurate diagnosis. Traditionally, pathologists or cytotechnologists are required to be on-site where the procedures are being performed. This can tie up valuable manpower for an extended period of time especially if it is a particular challenging case. The use of synchronous, real-time telepathology services will enable more procedurists to have access to ROSE and improve the diagnostic yield of tissue obtained [22].

It is extremely important that the local regulations and infrastructure are supportive of telemedicine alternatives. Before embarking on a telemedicine program, centres should craft their program aiming to maximize the quality of patient care whilst minimizing the risks of liability for healthcare programs. Considerations include:

1. Adequate training of the healthcare team and patient
2. Indemnity/insurance coverage for telemedicine
3. Whether the quality of information acquired during the teleconsult is adequate to formulate a diagnosis or treatment plan
4. Potential limitations to assessment of the patient, such as

   (a) Inability of the medical team to perform a physical examination
   (b) Lack of visual and other cues compared to an in-person consultation
   (c) Technological limitations (e.g. transmission delay, potential for data breach) [25]

Limitations that are relevant to the treatment of the patient should be openly disclosed and discussed so that patients understand the risks before agreeing to receiving care through telemedicine. Should care providers feel that adequate assessment of the patient via telemedicine is not possible, they should always recommend that the patient be seen in person at a clinic or Emergency Department [25].

As with any consult, adequate documentation and patient privacy remain of utmost importance and should not be neglected. The healthcare team should also be aware that such consults can also be easily recorded by patients even if in-program recording functions are turned off. Regardless of an individual's view on such surreptitious recordings, healthcare providers should be cognizant of the fact that these can be used as admissible evidence in future civil claims or disciplinary proceedings. It is prudent that the healthcare team continues to conduct themselves professionally on the assumption that every encounter is being recorded [25].

Technology has the potential to improve the patient experience and free up healthcare manpower to better optimize patient care. This can herald better multidisciplinary patient care, cost savings, increased patient access to treatment, clinical trials and education. With the appropriate focus on physician training, reimbursement and infrastructure development while addressing deficits inherent in the digital divide, telemedicine can be a powerful in the future of outpatient cancer care [23].

Outpatient Cancer Care in a Pandemic

The COVID19 Pandemic that began in early 2020 greatly impacted healthcare worldwide, not just cancer care. Apart from the obvious strain on healthcare resources, it has also had a significant impact on global economies and international travel. The COVID19 pandemic is not the first such disaster the world has faced, and will not be the last.

Considerations for cancer care that need to be undertaken in a pandemic are unique and aimed at addressing the negative effects it has on cancer treatment and research. Cancer patients and HSCT recipients are an especially vulnerable population who are at higher risks of complications from any pandemic illness and should take extra safety precautions. A retrospective analysis of 355 patients who died of COVID19 in Italy showed that 20% had active cancer [26]. Healthcare resource scarcity due to the influx of non-cancer patients into the healthcare system also disrupts the routine treatment of cancer and HSCT [27]. Serious and disruptive effects are also wrought upon the conduct of haematology and oncology clinical trials with reduction in recruitment, and delay in drug development timelines [28].

It is imperative during such pandemics that healthcare teams address the following issues:

1. Which specific populations are most at risk
2. Decisions for initiation or continuation of treatment, with careful balancing of risk/benefit
3. Cancer patient prioritization by anticipated outcomes [28]

Specific to the COVID19 pandemic, measures undertaken in the outpatient setting include:

1. Follow-up appointments by phone or telemedicine where possible
2. Prioritize oral or subcutaneous routes of drug delivery over infusional routes
3. Perform blood tests out of hospital
4. Home delivery of medications and administration of infusional medications at home if possible
5. Critical triaging of second opinions [28]
6. Cryopreservation of donor stem cells or arranging alternative sources (e.g. cord blood) for HSCT

While every pandemic and wide-scale disaster will present its own unique challenges, it is important for haematology and oncology units to be as well prepared as possible for such eventualities through the gleaning of knowledge from prior experiences. The COVID19 pandemic of 2020 has shown how disastrous and deadly the lack of preparation can be for any healthcare system, cancer care notwithstanding.

References

1. Sive J, Ardeshna KM, Cheesman S, le Grange F, Morris S, Nicholas C, Peggs K, Statham P, Goldstone AH. Hotel-based ambulatory care for complex cancer patients: a review of the University College London Hospital experience. Leuk Lymphoma. 2012;53(12):2397–404.
2. Joo E-H, Rha S-Y, Ahn JB, Kang H-Y. Economic and patient-reported outcomes of outpatient home-based versus inpatient hospital-based chemotherapy for patients with colorectal cancer. Support Care Cancer. 2010;19(7):971–8. https://doi.org/10.1007/s00520-010-0917-7.
3. Reid RM, Baran A, Friedberg JW, Phillips GL 2nd, Liesveld JL, Becker MW, Wedow L, Barr PM, Milner LA. Outpatient administration of BEAM conditioning prior to autologous stem cell transplantation for lymphoma is safe, feasible, and cost-effective. Cancer Med. 2016;5(11):3059–67.
4. Prip A, Møller KA, Nielsen DL, Jarden M, Olsen M-H, Danielsen AK. The patient–healthcare professional relationship and communication in the oncology outpatient setting. Cancer Nurs. 2018;41(5):E11–22. https://doi.org/10.1097/NCC.0000000000000533.
5. Towle EL, Barr TR, Hanley A, Kosty M, Williams S, Goldstein MA. Results of the ASCO study of collaborative practice arrangements. J Oncol Pract. 2011;7(5):278–82. https://doi.org/10.1200/JOP.2011.000385.
6. Reynolds RB, McCoy K. The role of Advanced Practice Providers in interdisciplinary oncology care in the United States. Chin Clin Oncol. 2016;5(3):44. https://doi.org/10.21037/cco.2016.05.01.
7. Williamson TS. The shift of oncology inpatient care to outpatient care: the challenge of retaining expert oncology nurses. Clin J Oncol Nurs. 2008;12(2):186–9. https://doi.org/10.1188/08.CJON.186-189.
8. Monas L, Toren O, Uziely B, Chinitz D. The oncology nurse coordinator: role perceptions of staff members and nurse coordinators. Isr J Health Policy Res. 2017;6(1):66. https://doi.org/10.1186/s13584-017-0186-8.
9. Thoma J, Zelkó R, Hankó B. The need for community pharmacists in oncology outpatient care: a systematic review. Int J Clin Pharm. 2016;38(4):855–62. https://doi.org/10.1007/s11096-016-0297-2.

10. Lamé G, Jouini O, Stal-Le Cardinal J. Outpatient chemotherapy planning: a literature review with insights from a case study. IIE Trans Healthc Syst Eng. 2016;6(3):127–39. https://doi.org/10.1080/19488300.2016.1189469.

11. Jagannath S, Vesole DH, Zhang M, et al. Feasibility and cost effectiveness of outpatient auto-transplants in multiple myeloma. Bone Marrow Transplant. 1997;20:445–50.

12. Seropian S, Nadkarni R, Jillella AP, et al. Neutropenic infections in 100 patients with non-Hodgkin's lymphoma or Hodgkin's disease treated with high-dose BEAM chemotherapy and peripheral blood progenitor cell transplant: out-patient treatment is a viable option. Bone Marrow Transplant. 1999;23:599–605.

13. McSweeney PA, Niederwieser D, Shizuru JA, Sandmaier BM, Molina AJ, Maloney DG, Chauncey TR, Gooley TA, Hegenbart U, Nash RA, Radich J, Wagner JL, Minor S, Appelbaum FR, Bensinger WI, Bryant E, Flowers ME, Georges GE, Grumet FC, Kiem HP, Torok-Storb B, Yu C, Blume KG, Storb RF. Hematopoietic cell transplantation in older patients with hematologic malignancies: replacing high-dose cytotoxic therapy with graft-versus-tumor effects. Blood. 2001;97(11):3390–400.

14. Trujillo EB, Claghorn K, Dixon SW, Hill EB, Braun A, Lipinski E, et al. Inadequate nutrition coverage in outpatient cancer centers: results of a national survey. J Oncol. 2019;2019(5):1–8. https://doi.org/10.1155/2019/7462940.

15. Mehnert A, Brahler E, Faller H, Harter M, Keller M, Schulz H, et al. Four-week prevalence of mental disorders in patients with cancer across major tumor entities. J Clin Oncol. 2014;32(31):3540–6. https://doi.org/10.1200/JCO.2014.56.0086. PMID: 25287821.

16. Liang B, Turkcan A, Ceyhan ME, Stuart K. Improvement of chemotherapy patient flow and scheduling in an outpatient oncology clinic. Int J Prod Res. 2015;53(24):7177–90. https://doi.org/10.1080/00207543.2014.988891.

17. Lau PKH, Watson MJ, Hasani A. Patients prefer chemotherapy on the same day as their medical oncology outpatient appointment. J Oncol Pract. 2014;10(6):e380–4. https://doi.org/10.1200/JOP.2014.001545.

18. Soh TIP, Tan YS, Hairom Z, Ibrahim M, Yao Y, Wong YP, et al. Improving wait times for elective chemotherapy through pre-preparation: a quality-improvement project at the National University Cancer Institute of Singapore. J Oncol Pract. 2015;11(1):e89–94. https://doi.org/10.1200/JOP.2014.000356.

19. Masselink IHJ, van der Mijden TLC, Litvak N, Vanberkel PT. Preparation of chemotherapy drugs: planning policy for reduced waiting times. Omega, Elsevier. 2012;40(2):181–7.

20. Coelho SM, Pinto CF, Calado RD, Silva MB. Process improvement in a cancer outpatient chemotherapy unit using lean healthcare. In: IFAC proceedings volumes, vol. 46. IFAC; 2015. p. 241–6. https://doi.org/10.3182/20130911-3-BR-3021.00047.

21. Lai L. Waiting time at National Cancer Centre reduced with RFID system. The Straits Times. 2013. Retrieved from https://www.straitstimes.com/singapore/waiting-time-at-national-cancer-centre-reduced-with-rfid-system.

22. Sirintrapun SJ, Lopez AM. Telemedicine in cancer care. Am Soc Clin Oncol Educ Book. 2018;38:540–5. https://doi.org/10.1200/EDBK_200141.

23. Yunus F, Gray S, Fox KC, Allen JW, Sachdev J, Merkel M, et al. The impact of telemedicine in cancer care. J Clin Oncol. 2009;27(15_suppl):e20508. https://doi.org/10.1200/jco.2009.27.15_suppl.e20508.

24. Wolfgang K. Telemedicine expands oncology care options. Oncol Times. 2019;41(8):13,19. https://doi.org/10.1097/01.COT.0000557852.06846.47.

25. En Ying K, Wei Munn M, Tee C, Hsu Hsien T. Covid-19 and issues facing the healthcare community: how can telemedicine help? April 23, 2020. Retrieved April 29, 2020, from https://www.allenandgledhill.com/sg/perspectives/articles/14781/sgkh-covid-19-and-issues-facing-the-healthcare-community-how-can-telemedicine-help.

26. Onder G, Rezza G, Brusaferro S. Case-fatality rate and characteristics of patients dying in relation to COVID-19 in Italy. JAMA. 2020;323(18):1775–6. https://doi.org/10.1001/jama.2020.4683.

27. Saini KS, de Las Heras B, de Castro J, Venkitaraman R, Poelman M, Srinivasan G, et al. Effect of the COVID-19 pandemic on cancer treatment and research. Lancet Haematol. 2020;7(6):e432–5. https://doi.org/10.1016/S2352-3026(20)30123-X.
28. van de Haar J, Hoes LR, Coles CE, et al. Caring for patients with cancer in the COVID-19 era. Nat Med. 2020;26(5):665–71. https://doi.org/10.1038/s41591-020-0874-8.

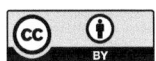

Chapter 5
The Infusion Center

Mohamed A. Kharfan-Dabaja

Introduction

Cancer remains a major public health problem worldwide. In the United States, cancer represents the second leading cause of death [1]. Availability of more effective supportive therapies, namely, new generation of antimicrobials, antiemetics, and hematopoietic growth factors, among others, coupled with emergence of novel antineoplastic agents, have facilitated administration of cancer treatments outside the hospital setting [2–4]. Moreover, a significant number of new targeted therapies for various cancers are more amenable to being offered in the outpatient infusion center setting owing to a better toxicity profile [5, 6]. Another factor driving increased utilization of infusion centers include a lower healthcare cost when compared to the inpatient hospital setting. For instance, receiving a cancer treatment in a hospital will definitely cost more than if it were administered in an infusion center for the same medication at the same dose and frequency. This is also the case for other supportive therapies.

Cancer treatments typically require multiple visits. The logistics can be exhausting for patients and their caregivers who are already under a lot of stress including physical, emotional, and financial strain, among others. There are times when visitors may be restricted at the discretion of nursing staff. Receiving a treatment in an infusion center is definitely more convenient than going to a hospital, considering the increased hassle and complexities associated with the latter. Infusion centers are purposely designed to provide a calm environment for people receiving chemotherapy and other types of infusions, hence resulting in an improved psychological well-being. Yet, presently the role of the infusion center transcends beyond

M. A. Kharfan-Dabaja (✉)
Division of Hematology-Oncology, Mayo Clinic, Jacksonville, FL, USA

Blood and Marrow Transplantation Program, Mayo Clinic, Jacksonville, FL, USA
e-mail: KharfanDabaja.Mohamed@mayo.edu

M. Aljurf et al. (eds.), *The Comprehensive Cancer Center*,
https://doi.org/10.1007/978-3-030-82052-7_5

antineoplastic treatment administration. Below, we highlight the main services provided by infusion centers.

Infusion Center Area

Generally, infusion areas comprise a mix of beds and recliner chairs which are assigned based on the needs of the patient and the type of treatment that they will be receiving. Other services include on-site cable television, computers, and Wi-Fi access. Also, with the advent of electronic health records the contemporary design of infusion center rooms incorporate a computer working station for added convenience and efficiency (Fig. 5.1). Infusion centers provide a multitude of services including but not limited to:

(a) Administration of blood products
(b) Intravenous biotherapies
(c) Chemotherapies: intravenous or subcutaneous
(d) Antimicrobial therapies
(e) Intravenous fluid including electrolytes replacement
(f) Other therapies

   (i) Bisphosphonates or similar therapies for bone protection
   (ii) Intravenous iron replacement therapy

(g) Nurse educators and library resources

Infusion centers allow providers to help patients better manage and control their disease and associated symptoms by providing a continuity of care throughout their medical need. By enhancing continuity of care, it improves patient compliance.

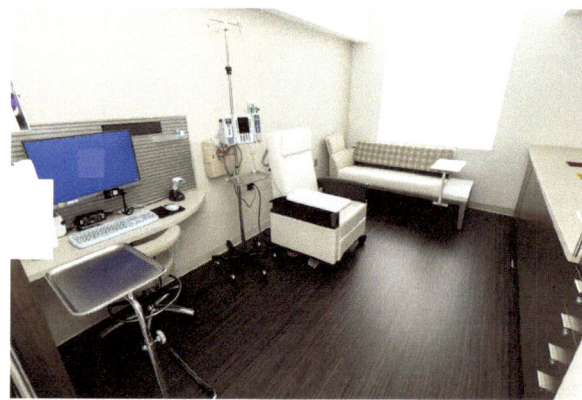

Fig. 5.1 Outpatient infusion center, Mayo Clinic, Jacksonville, FL, USA. (Used with permission of Mayo Foundation for Medical Education and Research, all rights reserved)

Infusion centers, in academic hospitals and even community-based setting, which are actively participating in research, do offer experimental therapy(ies) which encompass new drugs, or use existing drugs prescribed in new ways or on new diseases, among others. All medical and nursing staff are generally trained in oncology and clinical trial patient care. Clinical lab facilities are usually present on-site for proper specimen management. Most clinical trials, particularly phase 1 and 2 studies would also require presence of advanced cardiovascular life support certified personnel and equipment; for example, a defibrillator on-site in case patients develop untoward side effects to experimental therapies being administered. Pharmacists are also available on-site for the purpose of preparing and compounding antineoplastic agents; and to help determine the possibility of drug–drug interactions or to closely monitor administration of experimental therapies as part of clinical trials.

Staff

The team in a cancer center infusion facility consists of medical oncologists/hematologists, advanced practice providers, and certified oncology nurses who are available to help support your treatment needs in a safe manner. Other services that are available according to specific patients' needs include:

(a) Social workers
(b) Case managers
(c) Nutrition therapists/dietary counselors
(d) Health and wellness counselors
(e) Administrative staff to assist with insurance-related issues or referrals to other clinical services.

Other On-Site Services

Clinical labs: Presence of on-site clinical labs provides added convenience to the patient and allows administration of prescribed therapies in a more timely fashion. While the capabilities and level of sophistication varies among centers, these labs, at the minimum, should be able to offer a complete blood count with a differential and a comprehensive metabolic panel. In cancer centers that perform complex procedures like allogeneic hematopoietic cell transplantation (allo-HCT), these on-site labs may also have capabilities to measure blood titers of immune suppressants, among others.

Diagnostic imaging: In large cancer centers, patients are able to have basic diagnostic imaging in close proximity to the infusion center, generally within the same building. The level of complexity of diagnostic services provided varies among centers, but generally standard radiologic testing such as chest X-ray are generally readily available. It is important to keep in mind that there is no universal model for what diagnostic imaging services must be available in close proximity of an infusion center, and it would certainly depend on available financial resources and architectural design, among others.

Disease-specific support services: Owing to the different type of treatments offered at an infusion center, various support services are available. This includes but is not limited to physicians, nurses, and advanced practice providers specialized in various specialties such as infectious diseases, hematology, and medical oncology, among others. Also, for those patients receiving their first cycle of therapy, a lot of education about the potential side effect(s) of newly prescribed antineoplastic agents or potential drug–drug interactions are provided by nurses and/or specialized pharmacists. Disease-specific educational materials such as booklets are regularly available on-site to be shared with patients and caregivers.

Infusion Centers: Convenience and Potential Healthcare Cost Savings

Availability of infusion centers in the outpatient setting provides a smoother transition of care from the inpatient to the outpatient setting in patients who had completed induction antineoplastic therapies for diseases like acute myeloid leukemia, or complex procedures such as HCT, both autologous (auto-HCT) or allo-HCT, and other cellular therapies, namely, chimeric antigen receptor T (CAR T)-cell therapy in the hospital setting. Generally, patients who undergo these procedures are required to continue to be followed closely for few weeks in the case of auto-HCT and CAR T-cell therapy, or for longer time (typically, approx. 2–3 months) in allo-HCT recipients [7–9]. These patients are required to stay in the vicinity of the cancer center for close surveillance and needed clinical management. Among the clinical services provided to these patients include administration of intravenous fluids and electrolytes, antimicrobials, transfusion of blood products and certain antineoplastic therapies. Although there are no established standards for hours of operations, in some cases infusion centers provide extended hours and weekend day access.

The cost of health care is rising at an unsustainable rate in the United States, and it is expected to continue to rise because of population changes and the high cost of novel anti-cancer therapies, among other reasons [10, 11]. Availability of outpatient cancer infusion centers has the potential to reduce readmission rates to the inpatient hospital setting [12]. This is possible by providing services like transfusion of blood products, intravenous fluids, antimicrobials, and others, which traditionally need to be administered in the hospital. This results in a twofold benefit of not only preventing readmissions to the hospital, which is a national policy priority, but also providing aforementioned services at a lower cost.

Remaining Challenges

Cancer care is complex both logistically and operationally. Financial aspects related to the practice of oncology could be challenging owing to the very expensive cost of cancer drugs and the need to secure prior authorizations from third-party payers for certain therapies. This requirement can be at times problematic and could potentially affect the overall delivery of efficient and timely care. Also, during the COVID-19 pandemic caused by SARS-CoV-2, individual patient's decision needed to be made which could have resulted in delaying administration of chemotherapy. This has certainly been a learning lesson, and different oncology societies have developed guidelines on cancer care which will certainly help being better prepared for similar future events [13, 14].

Discussion

We described the major components required for successful operation of a cancer infusion center. The ultimate goals of a successful infusion center are to offer a patient-centered experience that improves the overall quality of delivered care at a sustainable cost. Beyond comfort and convenience, infusion centers are helpful in providing continuity of care, adherence to prescribed therapies, and administration of supportive therapies whenever indicated. This could have a beneficial effect on reducing readmissions to the hospital and improve patient satisfaction.

Conflicts of Interests   The author discloses consultancy for Pharmacyclics and Daiichi Sankyo.

References

1. Siegel RL, Miller KD, Jemal A. Cancer statistics, 2020. CA Cancer J Clin. 2020;70(1):7–30.
2. Herbrecht R, et al. Voriconazole versus amphotericin B for primary therapy of invasive aspergillosis. N Engl J Med. 2002;347(6):408–15.
3. Navari RM, Aapro M. Antiemetic prophylaxis for chemotherapy-induced nausea and vomiting. N Engl J Med. 2016;374(14):1356–67.
4. Bennett CL, et al. Colony-stimulating factors for febrile neutropenia during cancer therapy. N Engl J Med. 2013;368(12):1131–9.
5. Schmid P, et al. Pembrolizumab for early triple-negative breast cancer. N Engl J Med. 2020;382(9):810–21.

6. Zinzani PL, et al. Efficacy and safety of pembrolizumab in relapsed/refractory primary mediastinal large B-cell lymphoma (rrPMBCL): updated analysis of the KEYNOTE-170 phase 2 trial. Blood. 2017;130(Suppl 1):2833.
7. Kharfan-Dabaja MA, et al. Haematopoietic cell transplantation for blastic plasmacytoid dendritic cell neoplasm: a North American multicentre collaborative study. Br J Haematol. 2017;179(5):781–9.
8. Neelapu SS, et al. Axicabtagene ciloleucel CAR T-cell therapy in refractory large B-cell lymphoma. N Engl J Med. 2017;377(26):2531–44.
9. Schuster SJ, et al. Tisagenlecleucel in adult relapsed or refractory diffuse large B-cell lymphoma. N Engl J Med. 2019;380(1):45–56.
10. Mariotto AB, et al. Projections of the cost of cancer care in the United States: 2010-2020. J Natl Cancer Inst. 2011;103(2):117–28.
11. Marsland T, et al. Reducing cancer costs and improving quality through collaboration with payers: a proposal from the Florida society of clinical oncology. J Oncol Pract. 2010;6(5):265–9.
12. Montero AJ, et al. Reducing unplanned medical oncology readmissions by improving outpatient care transitions: a process improvement project at the Cleveland Clinic. J Oncol Pract. 2016;12(5):e594–602.
13. Burki TK. Cancer guidelines during the COVID-19 pandemic. Lancet Oncol. 2020;21(5):629–30.
14. Tian J, et al. Clinical characteristics and risk factors associated with COVID-19 disease severity in patients with cancer in Wuhan, China: a multicentre, retrospective, cohort study. Lancet Oncol. 2020;21(7):893–903.

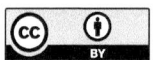

Chapter 6
Proposal for Establishing a New Radiotherapy Facility

Mohamed Aldehaim and Jack Phan

Introduction

Cancer is a significant cause of morbidity and mortality. As per multiple cancer registries, the incidence of cancer is increasing worldwide. The highest increase is observed among low- and middle-income countries [1]. Radiotherapy is a crucial and cost-effective component of cancer care and can be utilized in the definitive, adjuvant, and palliative settings. Radiation therapy has been shown to increase overall survival in many types of locally advanced cancers. Around half of all cancer patients will receive radiation treatment at some point during their course of treatment [2, 3].

A radiotherapy facility is an integral component of a multidisciplinary cancer center. Along with surgical intervention and chemotherapy, radiotherapy is crucial and needed in designing a cancer care facility. Once the decision to establish a radiotherapy facility has been made, careful strategic planning is needed to ensure alignment with the cancer center's overall mission and goals concerning available resources. Recruitment of skilled clinicians and personnel is critical to ensure safe and high-quality patient care. Coordination and monitoring of the planning and timelines are critical to a successful project, especially when resources are limited. The professional team required to design, construct, and commission a radiotherapy facility needs to be in a multidisciplinary sitting from various background [4].

This chapter presents an overview of radiotherapy's value in treating the most common clinically indicated malignancies worldwide. We aim to present a proposal

M. Aldehaim
Department of Radiation Oncology, King Faisal Specialist Hospital & Research Center, Riyadh, Saudi Arabia

J. Phan (✉)
Department of Radiation Oncology, The University of Texas MD Anderson Cancer Center, Houston, TX, USA
e-mail: jphan@mdanderson.org

© The Author(s) 2022
M. Aljurf et al. (eds.), *The Comprehensive Cancer Center*,
https://doi.org/10.1007/978-3-030-82052-7_6

to assess the radiotherapy facility's clinical, infrastructure, and resources need while establishing a new radiotherapy facility.

Population Description

Determining the need for radiation therapy requires in-depth knowledge of the population demographics, cancer incidence, and national disease burden estimates with precise projections for the future [5]. Establishing cancer registries is essential for estimating the community's clinical needs, developing clinical pathways, and implementing research programs. Further forecasts regarding anticipated radiotherapy capacity and use (number of radiation courses and fractions per course for each cancer type, as well as the amount of potential retreatment) should also be estimated [6]. These steps are unique for each nation and country. In the countries where these variables are not measured, the International Agency for Research on Cancer (IARC) provides the best estimate of crude incidence, Table 6.1 and Fig. 6.1.

Needs Assessment

The target population is subdivided into various tumor sites. According to multiple cancer registries, most treated cases will include breast, prostate, lung, and colorectal cancers. Data from Australia [7] indicates that a curative radiotherapy course

Table 6.1 World Cancer Statistics per International Agency for Research on Cancer, World Health Organization 2018

Summary statistic 2018			
	Males	Females	Both sexes
Population	3,850,719,284	3,782,099,828	7,632,819,272
Number of new cancer cases	9,456,418	8,622,539	18,078,957
Age-standardized incidence rate (world)	218.6	182.6	197.9
Risk of developing cancer before the age of 75 years (%)	22.4	18.3	20.2
Number of cancer deaths	5,385,640	4,169,387	9,555,027
Age-standardized mortality rate (world)	122.7	83.1	101.1
Risk of dying from cancer before the age of 75 years (%)	12.7	8.7	10.6
5-year prevalent cases	21,014,830	22,826,472	43,841,302
Top 5 most frequent cancers excluding nonmelanoma skin cancer (ranked by cases)	Lung	Breast	Lung
	Prostate	Colorectum	Breast
	Colorectum	Lung	Colorectum
	Stomach	Cervix uteri	Prostate
	Liver	Thyroid	Stomach

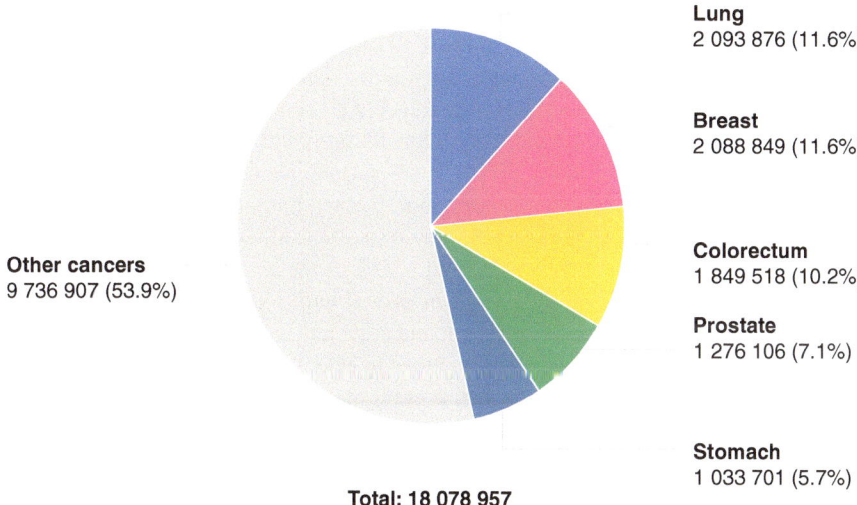

Fig. 6.1 Number of new cancer cases in 2018 by sites, both sexes, all ages. (Source: International Agency for Research on Cancer, World Health Organization 2018)

requires an average of 22 fractions and a palliative course 4 fractions; thus, the total average would be 18 fractions per the first course. The average linear accelerator (linac) treats four to five patients per hour, so the total linac utilization will depend on the total number of hours per day that the machine is active.

In the developed world, most breast cancer (approximately 95%) cases present at potentially curative early stage or locally advanced cases. Evidence of treating breast cases with hypofractionation is well established [8] and widely utilized worldwide.

Similarly, for prostate cancer, due to screening, the majority of cases will present at an early stage (low-risk disease). Treatment options for low-risk prostate cancer include active surveillance (standard of care), radical prostatectomy, external beam radiotherapy, or brachytherapy. It is estimated that 60% of these cases will receive external beam radiation treatment, either definitively or in the early salvage setting, during their disease trajectories. The majority of cases are treated with conventional fractionation (although early salvage radiation usually requires a lower radiation dosage) [9]. Hypofractionation is increasingly an attractive option and often delivered in 20 fractions [10] or fewer. Recently, there is growing evidence of ultra-hypofractionation with seven or fewer fractions that have been utilized in many cancer centers [11].

Lung cancers can be categorized into non-small cell lung cancer (NSCLC) and small cell lung cancer (SCLC), which require different radiotherapy treatment protocols. For NSCLC, stages 1 and 2 comprise 30% of presenting cases, and some of them (medically inoperable) will be treated with curative intent Stereotactic Body Radiotherapy (SBRT). It is estimated that a small percentage will receive SBRT with five or fewer fractions for peripherally located tumors and eight to ten fractions for centrally located one [12]. Approximately, 45% of NSCLC cases present at stage III and are treated with concurrent chemoradiation [13]. For SCLC, which comprises

~15% of all lung cancer cases, both limited and extensive stage presentations are considered. For limited-stage SCLC (33% of cases), the radiation treatment is thoracic radiation with 30 fractions twice daily with at least 6 h apart [14] to follow with prophylactic cranial radiation in 10 fractions [15]. For extensive-stage SCLC (66% of cases), the standard treatment is a systemic therapy, and the responder will require consolidative thoracic radiation with [16] +/− prophylactic cranial radiation [17].

In the category of colorectal cancers, radiotherapy has a more limited role except for rectal cancers, where radiation treatment is often utilized. Rectal cancers comprise of ~28% of colorectal cancers, and ~20% of rectal cancers are metastatic at presentation. The remaining 80% is often treated with long-course chemoradiation [18], which is typical in the neoadjuvant and adjuvant setting. Another alternative is short-course radiotherapy, with five fractions in selected cases.

For endometrial cancer, most cases present at an early stage and need observation or vault brachytherapy in an adjuvant setting. However, assuming at most, 30% of endometrial cancers will require external beam radiation. This includes medically inoperable and adjuvant treatment cases treated with 25 fractions [19]. Approximately 60% of cervical cancers present between stage IB2 and stage IVA and require external beam radiation as part of treatment. The most common prescription is 25 fractions [20]. Approximately 40% of esophageal cancers present at a curable stage, requiring on average concurrent chemoradiation [21].

Palliative cases constitute a significant radiation oncology workload component, and up to 50% of all oncology cases may receive palliative intent treatment. This includes new patients presenting with the metastatic and non-curable disease, and previously treated patients who have developed a non-curable recurrence. The majority of palliative intent treatments constitute radiotherapy for bone metastases, brain metastases, and spinal cord compression. For bone metastases, the most common prescription is single or a few fractions. For spinal cord compression, the most common prescription is ten or fewer fractions. For brain metastases, the main treatment options include fractionated whole-brain radiation or stereotactic radiosurgery (SRS) with single fraction doses ranging from 15 to 24 Gy depending on the target's size [22].

Head and neck cancers and sarcomas typically require the services of surgical oncologists with highly specialized training. There is existing evidence that supports that the outcomes for head and neck cancers [23], sarcomas [24], and bladder cancers [25] are significantly better in tertiary high-volume centers with specialized care in these areas. Similarly, pediatric oncology is highly subspecialized and requires input and management from multiple disciplines.

Brachytherapy

This section focuses on the use of brachytherapy to treat prostate, endometrial, and cervical cancers. For prostate cancer, brachytherapy can be used as monotherapy for low-risk and intermediate-risk patients, or in combination with external beam radiation therapy (EBRT) as a form of dose escalation for selected intermediate-risk and

Intermediate risk

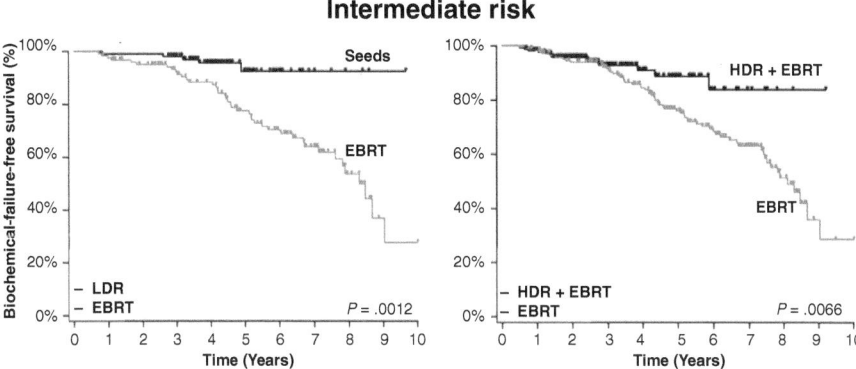

Fig. 6.2 Kaplan-Meier curves comparing propensity score-matched patients receiving external beam radiation therapy (EBRT) versus brachytherapy (BT) for intermediate-risk patients. (Smith et al. [27])

high-risk patients. Brachytherapy with either permanent implants (low dose rate [LDR]) or temporary implants (high dose rate [HDR]) has become an integral component of radiation therapy with excellent oncological outcome [26]. There is well-established evidence suggesting that low and intermediate-risk prostate cancer patients who are treated with brachytherapy have superior outcomes compared to EBRT in terms of better biochemical failure-free survival (e.g., PROCARS Database where 7974 prostate cancer patients managed at four Canadian institutions 1994–2010 Fig. 6.2) [27]. This evidence supports the increased utilization of brachytherapy treatment.

The general rationale for using brachytherapy is as follows:

1. Dose escalation is required to maximize cancer control.
2. Brachytherapy enables increased dose delivery to the target and sparing of adjacent healthy tissues.
3. The low α/β ratio of prostate cancer provides a radiobiological rationale for HDR brachytherapy.
4. There is a substantial body of clinical evidence to support the use of prostate brachytherapy.

Many cancer centers plan to use only HDR brachytherapy instead of permanent implants LDR as there is a dosimetric and practical rationale for this. Because dose optimization with HDR brachytherapy is performed after placement of catheters, HDR enables more consistent target coverage and excellent dose uniformity, resulting in a lower dose to the urethra and rectum when compared to permanent seed implants [28]. Currently, there is no clinical evidence to suggest that HDR brachytherapy is inferior to LDR brachytherapy. Thus, offering HDR brachytherapy alone is a cost-effective solution without compromising clinical efficacy when resources are limited.

It is estimated that ~13–15% of total prostate cancer patients will eventually receive brachytherapy (LDR or HDR) alone or combined with EBRT. The suggested dose and fractionation schemes are detailed in Table 6.2.

Table 6.2 Suggested dose and fractionation for HDR brachytherapy in prostate cancer

	Single fraction boost (before EBRT)	HDR monotherapy	Focal salvage
Dose fractionation	15 Gy/1 F	19 Gy/1 F (worse outcome) Or 13.5 Gy/2 F (1 week apart)	13.5 Gy/2 F (1 week apart)

Table 6.3 Suggested dose and fractionation for HDR brachytherapy in endometrial cancer

Scenario	External beam dose	HDR dose per fraction	Number of fractions
Adjuvant with EBRT	45 Gy/25	5.5 Gy to 0.5 cm	2
Sole adjuvant	0	7 Gy to 0.5 cm	3
Recurrence with EBRT	45 Gy/25 50.4 Gy/28	7 Gy to 0.5 cm 6 Gy to 0.5 cm	2 2
Recurrence following previous RT	0	7 Gy to 0.5 cm	3

We estimate that a high number of patients will be diagnosed with endometrial cancer. The majority of these cancers are seen in postmenopausal women, with a median age of 60 years. The majority of them will be early stage disease and require surgical intervention with a total abdominal hysterectomy and bilateral salpingo-oophorectomy (TAH-BSO). We estimate that at most we will treat one-third with vaginal vault brachytherapy either alone or in combination with external beam radiation therapy. Each patient will require two to three fractions of treatment. Patients are routinely booked for three insertions to allow the additional dose to be given if there is an incomplete response after two insertions.

There are three sets of vaginal vault applicators depending on size (small, medium, and large). Most utilize cylindrical applicators (various diameters (20–40 mm) and lengths (2.5–10 cm)) with a dome cylinder at the top and with one central channel or two to three channels in different configurations. The suggested dose and fractionation schemes are detailed in Table 6.3.

It is well established that HDR brachytherapy is an essential component of cervical cancer management. It has been estimated that 70% of these patients will be candidates for HDR brachytherapy. There is growing evidence that better oncological outcomes can be achieved with the utilization of MRI guidance. As per the consensus of the Brachytherapy in Cervical Cancer Expert Working Group (BCCEWG) Panel of the Cancer Care Ontario (CCO) meeting in 2009 [29], MRI was strongly recommended for delineation of target volumes and planning. The meeting concluded that CT provided acceptable but significantly inferior soft-tissue delineation and, in many cases, could not accurately delineate the target volumes. As per BCCEWG, cervical Brachytherapy also requires that it should only be done at centers with direct access to appropriate gynecological expertise for multidisciplinary patient assessment. The suggested dose and fractionation schemes are detailed in Table 6.4.

Table 6.4 Suggested dose and fractionation for brachytherapy prescription for cervical cancer

Scenario	External beam dose	HDR dose per fraction	Number of fractions
Standard prescription	45 Gy/25 + parametrial boost	5.5 Gy to point A	5
Alternative prescription for patients requiring fewer HDR fractions	45 Gy/25 + parametrial boost	8 Gy to point A	3

Equipment

This section describes the required equipment for delivering both external beam radiation and brachytherapy. A radiotherapy center aiming at treating an average of 1000 patients/year need to be equipped with at least a single-photon energy unit, a brachytherapy afterloader (ideally for high dose-rate brachytherapy), a full range of applicators, a simulator, preferably a CT simulator, a computerized treatment planning system (TPS), patient immobilization devices, and a beam measurement and quality assurance (QA) equipment [30].

External Beam Radiotherapy

For a resource-limited area, the decision to use a cobalt-60 unit or a linear accelerator (linac) for radiotherapy depends on various factors. The use of linacs in developing countries is increasing [31]. With good infrastructure and reliable power supply, a linac is preferred, although curative and effective radiation treatments are possible with a cobalt-60 unit. Linacs can generate electron treatment beams that can be used to treat skin cancers. However, linacs require more frequent quality assurance that needs to be carried out by a medical physicist.

Most newer facilities are equipped with high-energy linacs with intensity-modulated radiation therapy (IMRT), volumetric arc therapy (VMAT), and image-guided radiation therapy (IGRT) capabilities. This will require a careful review of deliverables, functionality, technical specifications, and cost of all commercially available linacs. It is crucial to evaluate the quality of the manufacturer's service and technical support that they will provide.

Linacs will have different energies, with 6 MV photon beams and 15–18 MV photon beams as the more commonly used energies. There is no anticipated need for 25 MV capability because the uniformity produced by 18 MV photons over targets is generally deemed sufficient while yielding less neutron production and, therefore, requiring less shielding. Further, some manufacturers no longer provide a 25 MV photon beam as a standard option. Installing a linac with 25 MV photons will only increase the price of the unit with no anticipated great benefit for the clinic. Stereotactic radiation and ablative treatments can be performed on the linac, Gamma

Knife, or Cyberknife systems. There will be a need for a CT simulation unit which can be shared between the external beam radiation and brachytherapy programs.

Brachytherapy

There will be a need for a dedicated HDR brachytherapy suite with a treatment room and control area. The brachytherapy treatment room contains a mini operating theatre equipped with the following:

- A Remote afterloader
- An in-room radiation detector and check source
- Audiovisual communication systems
- A securely locked door and door interlock
- A multiple-position patient procedure table
- A mobile ultrasound machine for guidance
- Emergency crash cart and recovery equipment
- Survey meter
- An anesthesia area with patient monitoring equipment
- An operating room procedure light
- A sink and scrub area
- Emergency shut-off buttons

Both Co-60 and Ir-192 are commonly used as sources in HDR brachytherapy; however, Ir-192 is usually selected as the radiation source to be used for the remote afterloader system due to lower photon energy and advantages it offers with regard to radiation protection. For example, the use of Ir-192 results in the amount of concrete required to be cut in half compared to Co-60.

An adjacent control area will allow for safe monitoring of the brachytherapy procedure and patient. Cameras will be needed for patient observation. Intercom facilities between the treatment room and control area are required to permit direct communication with the patient during the treatment. There will be dedicated computers and planning workstation in the control room.

Recovery area [32, 33]

- One anesthesiologist need to be present in the facility until such time that the last surgical patient of the day is deemed fully conscious.
- A fully qualified registered two nurses need to be present in the room. They must know and be in charge of the equipment, critical supplies, personnel assignments, and duties.
- Two fully equipped recovery beds. There should be curtains or screens to allow privacy.
- Space allocated per bed/trolley should be at least 9 m^2. There must be easy access to the patient's head.
- Adequate space to allow the transport of patients and movement of personnel. A continuous oxygen delivery system must be in place.

- All necessary medical equipment from monitoring, suction, and resuscitation equipment must be available.
- The emergency power source must be available, which will provide adequate lighting essential area lighting, and have the capacity to operate all necessary equipment.

Commissioning

Once the equipment is acquired from vendors, it will be subject to acceptance testing where tests and measurements will be performed to ensure that the equipment of software meets the specifications set by the manufacturer. The manufacturer will indicate the acceptance testing protocol, and the testing process will be jointly carried out by the installation technicians and medical physicists. Each facility needs to have the necessary equipment for acceptance testing, which might include: a 3D water phantom scanner, ion chambers, electrometer X-ray films, and film laser scanner. The American Association of Physicists in Medicine (AAPM) makes available useful task group reports (TG-35, TG-40, and TG-43) that provide detailed information about linacs safety and quality assurance.

Room Shielding

Design of the radiation treatment room shielding incorporated consideration of As Low As Reasonably Achievable (ALARA) principles, International Atomic Energy Agency (IAEA) Safety Standard Series, National Council on Radiation Protection and Measurements (NCRP), and American Association of Physicists in Medicine (AAPM) corresponding reports and the requirements set by different Safety Commissions, which mandates the maximum allowed limits of radiation exposure to occupants adjacent to the treatment rooms. These limits depend on whether or not those occupants would be considered nuclear energy workers (e.g., radiation therapists) or members of the public (e.g., patient family members, administrative staff). Important factors influencing the room shielding requirements and, therefore, corresponding cost include but are not limited to the expected workload of the unit (output in dose (Gy) per year), maximum expected dose rates per fraction, conventional or specialized treatment protocols, and associated fractionation (e.g., stereotactic body radiation therapy (SBRT)) and a number of palliative fractions and expected dose.

Careful selection of treatment room placement can help save cost by aligning the rooms such that walls requiring more shielding are shared (e.g., primary walls) and preventing most walls from being adjacent to public areas (e.g., by having the bunkers underground where some walls are lined by the earth and having treatment areas aligned such that most do not border a public waiting area).

Radiotherapy Staffing

The core professional team in radiotherapy consists of radiation oncologists, radiation therapists, dosimetrists, and medical physicists supported by nursing, administration, and various medical officers.

Personnel

To best serve the population, and based on the proposed size of the facility with linacs and brachytherapy unit, we can anticipate the need for radiation oncologists (ROs). According to the Cancer Care Ontario (CCO), the number of ROs required at any radiation center is consistent regardless of the size of the center and is 1.8–2 ROs per linac. Many community radiation centers operated within that framework. To run the linacs and an additional brachytherapy unit, we propose using a factor of two ROs per linac. A 0.5 Full-Time Equivalent (FTE) anesthesiologist is required for Brachytherapy, and 1 FTE medical oncologist for concurrent chemoradiation.

Based on the proposed number of concurrent clinics, we also anticipate the need for a number of dedicated nurses. Those would be used to see patients coming for clinic appointments, for radiation review clinic, for the brachytherapy unit, to take calls from patients and other healthcare providers, to run the chemotherapy suite, and float nurses. There will be a need for clinic coordinators to help with patient flow. The facility will need radiation therapists to help run the facility. Generally, four therapists are needed per linac. Two would be required to run the CT sim and two more for the brachytherapy suite. An additional dosimetrist would be dedicated to radiation planning.

Other support staff required would include administrative assistants for the ROs, administrative assistants to check patients in for CT sim or radiation treatments, and janitorial staff.

Quality Assurance

The responsibility for quality assurance and safety falls on every individual working at the radiotherapy facility, including radiation therapists, physicists, and radiation oncologists. In this section, some of the planned quality assurance activities for radiation oncologists and physicists will be discussed.

Physics: Equipment-specific quality assurance will be performed on all treatment equipment and software. Regular and continuous QA testing for equipment will be necessary to ensure safe and correct functioning. A written equipment quality control program must specify the required policies and procedures:

1. Parameters to be tested or the tests to be performed
2. Instruments to be used to perform the tests
3. Test setup (geometry, etc.)
4. Frequency of the tests
5. Individuals responsible for testing
6. Expected results or values
7. Tolerance level
8. Action to be taken when tolerance is exceeded

QA procedures for treatment machines will be performed on a daily, monthly, and annual basis using the guidelines and recommendations specified in the TG-45 report "AAPM code of practice for radiotherapy accelerators: Report of AAPM Radiation Therapy Task Group No. 45". The radiation therapists will perform daily machine QA, whereas the monthly and annual QA procedures will be the responsibility of the physicists. QA will mandate compliance with the specific requirements for remote afterloading units of the HDR brachytherapy unit.

Physicists will also be responsible for "chart checks" before delivery of 20% of the total dose, where a review of the prescription and treatment plan will be performed along with an independent MU calculation. There will also be a weekly physics chart check to ensure that the treatment is delivered as intended.

Oncologists: Oncologists will participate in weekly tumor board conferences where there will be input from surgeons and medical oncologists, and other medical doctors for the management of difficult or challenging cases. Usually, each site will require two oncologists' practice in that specific area, so that peer review of plans can be performed. Each section will have dedicated weekly quality assurance rounds where this process can take place. Usually, the quality assurance rounds will require the presence of at least two oncologists, one physicist, and two radiation therapists.

Timeline

A typical timeline of approximately a few years from the time of approval to the time when patients can first be treated is reasonable. The proposed timeline would break down as follows:

1. Commissioning design, engineering firms, architectural plans (6–12 months)
2. Facility and bunker construction (1–2 years)
3. Install linacs, CT, brachytherapy equipment (6–12 months)
4. Get clinic space up and running (3–6 months)
5. Training for ROs, physicists, planners (3–6 months)

Table 6.5 Estimation of the cost of brachytherapy suite (please note as these values might vary significantly depending on regions)

Parameter	Low end	High end
HDR device	$250K	$350K
Applicator	$50K	$100K
OR table	$35K	$75K
Vault	$40K	$80K
US	$20K	$75K
Anesthesia	$50K	$100K
Planning system	$150K	$200K
Construction	$50K	$70K

Table 6.6 Staffing costs for the proposed radiation therapy facility (please note as these values might vary significantly depending on regions)

Staff	Cost per FTE ($)
Radiation oncologists	180,000
Other physicians (anesthesia, medical oncology)	180,000
Physicists	135,000
Nursing	65,000
Radiation therapists	80,000
Information technologists	80,000
Administrative assistants	50,000
Janitorial staff	30,000

Budget

The anticipated life span of technology is 10 years. The brachytherapy suite costs are estimated in Table 6.5.

In terms of personnel, the estimated salaries are drawn from the literature from Europe and converted to dollars [34]. Note that base salaries are included for radiation oncologists and not the fee for service aspect. The staffing costs are estimated in Table 6.6.

Conclusion

Establishing a new radiotherapy facility is a complicated and costly process that required careful planning, understanding of the local disease burden, infrastructure, and multimodality expertise. Each step has many obstacles and challenges. The people, time, and money commitment can be substantial but rewarding and reduce cancer patients' suffering.

References

1. Farmer P, Frenk J, Knaul FM, et al. Expansion of cancer care and control in countries of low and middle income: a call to action. Lancet. 2010;376:1186–93.
2. Barton MB, Frommer M, Shafiq J. Role of radiotherapy in cancer control in low-income and middle-income countries. Lancet Oncol. 2006;7:584–95.
3. Delaney GP, Barton MB. Evidence-based estimates of the demand for radiotherapy. Clin Oncol (R Coll Radiol). 2015;27:70–6.
4. International Atomic Energy Agency (IAEA). Radiotherapy facilities: master planning and concept design considerations. IAEA Human Health Reports No. 10. 2014.
5. Efstathiou JA, Heunis M, Karumekayi T, Makufa R, Bvochora-Nsingo M, Gierga DP, Suneja G, Grover S, Kasese J, Mmalane M, Moffat H, von Paleske A, Makhema J, Dryden-Peterson S. Establishing and delivering quality radiation therapy in resource-constrained settings: the story of Botswana. Oncologia. 2016;34(1):27–35. https://doi.org/10.1200/JCO.2015.62.8413.
6. Zubizarreta EH, Fidarova E, Healy B, Rosenblatt E. Need for radiotherapy in low and middle-income countries – the silent crisis continues. Clin Oncol (R Coll Radiol). 2015;27:107–14.
7. IIAMR and CCORE. Review of optimal radiotherapy utilisation rates. Liverpool, NSW: Ingham Institute for Applied Medical Research (IIAMR) – Collaboration for Cancer Outcomes Research and Evaluation (CCORE); 2013.
8. Whelan TJ, Pignol J-P, Levine MN, Julian JA, MacKenzie R, Parpia S, Shelley W, Grimard L, Bowen J, Lukka H, Perera F, Fyles A, Schneider K, Gulavita S, Freeman C. Long-term results of hypofractionated radiation therapy for breast cancer. N Engl J Med. 2010;362(6):513–20.
9. Hamdy FC, Donovan JL, Lane JA, Mason M, Metcalfe C, Holding P, Davis M, Peters TJ, Turner EL, Martin RM, Oxley J, Robinson M, Staffurth J, Walsh E, Bollina P, Catto J, Doble A, Doherty A, Gillatt D, Kockelbergh R, Kynaston H, Paul A, Powell P, Prescott S, Rosario DJ, Rowe E, Neal DE, ProtecT Study Group. 10-Year outcomes after monitoring, surgery, or radiotherapy for localized prostate cancer. N Engl J Med. 2016;375(15):1415–24.
10. Dearnaley D, Syndikus I, Mossop H, Khoo V, Birtle A, Bloomfield D, Graham J, Kirkbride P, Logue J, Malik Z, Money-Kyrle J, O'Sullivan JM, Panades M, Parker C, Patterson H, Scrase C, Staffurth J, Stockdale A, Tremlett J, Bidmead M, Mayles H, Naismith O, South C, Gao A, Cruickshank C, Hassan S, Pugh J, Griffin C, Hall E, CHHiP Investigators. Conventional versus hypofractionated high-dose intensity-modulated radiotherapy for prostate cancer: 5-year outcomes of the randomized, non-inferiority, phase 3 CHHiP trial. Lancet Oncol. 2016;17(8):1047–60.
11. Jackson WC, Silva J, Hartman HE, Dess RT, Kishan AU, Beeler WH, Gharzai LA, Jaworski EM, Mehra R, Hearn JWD, Morgan TM, Salam SS, Cooperberg MR, Mahal BA, Soni PD, Kaffenberger S, Nguyen PL, Desai N, Feng FY, Zumsteg ZS, Spratt DE. Stereotactic body radiation therapy for localized prostate cancer: a systematic review and meta-analysis of over 6,000 patients treated on prospective studies. Int J Radiat Oncol Biol Phys. 2019;104(4):778–89. https://doi.org/10.1016/j.ijrobp.2019.03.051.
12. Timmerman RD, Hu C, Michalski JM, Bradley JC, Galvin J, Johnstone DW, Choy H. Long-term results of stereotactic body radiation therapy in medically inoperable stage I non-small cell lung cancer. JAMA Oncol. 2018;4(9):1287–8. https://doi.org/10.1001/jamaoncol.2018.1258.
13. Bradley JD, Paulus R, Komaki R, Masters G, Blumenschein G, Schild S, Bogart J, Hu C, Forster K, Magliocco A, Kavadi V, Garces YI, Narayan S, Iyengar P, Robinson C, Wynn RB, Koprowski C, Meng J, Beitler J, Gaur R, Curran W Jr, Choy H. Standard-dose versus high-dose conformal radiotherapy with concurrent and consolidation carboplatin plus paclitaxel with or without cetuximab for patients with stage IIIA or IIIB non-small-cell lung cancer (RTOG 0617): a rerandomized two-by-two factorial phase 3 study. Lancet Oncol. 2015;16(2):187–99. https://doi.org/10.1016/S1470-2045(14)71207-0. Epub 2015 Jan 16.
14. Turrisi AT 3rd, Kim K, Blum R, Sause WT, Livingston RB, Komaki R, Wagner H, Aisner S, Johnson DH. Twice-daily compared with once-daily thoracic radiotherapy in limited

small-cell lung cancer treated concurrently with cisplatin and etoposide. N Engl J Med. 1999;340(4):265–71.

15. Aupérin A, Arriagada R, Pignon JP, Le Péchoux C, Gregor A, Stephens RJ, Kristjansen PE, Johnson BE, Ueoka H, Wagner H, Aisner J. Prophylactic cranial irradiation for patients with small-cell lung cancer in complete remission. Prophylactic Cranial Irradiation Overview Collaborative Group. N Engl J Med. 1999;341(7):476–84.

16. Slotman BJ, van Tinteren H, Praag JO, Knegjens JL, El Sharouni SY, Hatton M, Keijser A, Faivre-Finn C, Senan S. Use of thoracic radiotherapy for extensive-stage small-cell lung cancer: a phase 3 randomized controlled trial. Lancet. 2015;385(9962):36–42. https://doi. org/10.1016/S0140-6736(14)61085-0. Epub 2014 Sept 14.

17. Slotman B, Faivre-Finn C, Kramer G, Rankin E, Snee M, Hatton M, Postmus P, Collette L, Musat E, Suresh S, EORTC Radiation Oncology Group and Lung Cancer Group. Prophylactic cranial irradiation in extensive small-cell lung cancer. N Engl J Med. 2007;357(7):664–72. https://doi.org/10.1056/NEJMoa071780.

18. Sauer R, Becker H, Hohenberger W, Rödel C, Wittekind C, Fietkau R, Martus P, Tschmelitsch J, Hager E, Hess CF, Karstens J-H, Liersch T, Schmidberger H, Raab R, German Rectal Cancer Study Group. Preoperative versus postoperative chemoradiotherapy for rectal cancer. N Engl J Med. 2004;351(17):1731–40. https://doi.org/10.1056/NEJMoa040694.

19. Creutzberg CL, Nout RA, Lybeert MLM, Wárlám-Rodenhuis CC, Jobsen JJ, Mens J-WM, Lutgens LCHW, Pras E, van de Poll-Franse LV, van Putten WLJ, PORTEC Study Group. Fifteen-year radiotherapy outcomes of the randomized PORTEC-1 trial for endometrial carcinoma. Int J Radiat Oncol Biol Phys. 2011;81(4):e631–8. https://doi.org/10.1016/j. ijrobp.2011.04.013. Epub 2011 June 2.

20. Landoni F, Colombo A, Milani R, Placa F, Zanagnolo V, Mangioni C. Randomized study between radical surgery and radiotherapy for the treatment of stage IB-IIA cervical cancer: 20-year update. J Gynecol Oncol. 2017;28(3):e34. https://doi.org/10.3802/jgo.2017.28.e34. Epub 2017 Feb 24.

21. Joel S, van Lanschot JJB, Hulshof MCCM, van Hagen P, van Berge Henegouwen MI, Wijnhoven BPL, van Laarhoven HWM, Nieuwenhuijzen GAP, Hospers GAP, Bonenkamp JJ, Cuesta MA, Blaisse RJB, Busch ORC, Ten Kate FJW, Creemers G-JM, Punt CJA, Plukker JTM, Verheul HMW, Spillenaar Bilgen EJ, van Dekken H, van der Sangen MJC, Rozema T, Biermann K, Beukema JC, Piet AHM, van Rij CM, Reinders JG, Tilanus HW, Steyerberg EW, van der Gaast A, CROSS Study Group. Neoadjuvant chemoradiotherapy plus surgery versus surgery alone for oesophageal or junctional cancer (CROSS): long-term results of a randomised controlled trial. Lancet Oncol. 2015;16(9):1090–8. https://doi.org/10.1016/ S1470-2045(15)00040-6. Epub 2015 Aug 5.

22. Shaw E, Scott C, Souhami L, Dinapoli R, Kline R, Loeffler J, Farnan N. Single dose radiosurgical treatment of recurrent previously irradiated primary brain tumors and brain metastases: final report of RTOG protocol 90-05. Int J Radiat Oncol Biol Phys. 2000;47(2):291–8. https:// doi.org/10.1016/s0360-3016(99)00507-6.

23. Corry J, Peters LJ, Rischin D. Impact of center size and experience on outcomes in head and neck cancer. J Clin Oncol. 2015;33(2):138–40. https://doi.org/10.1200/JCO.2014.58.2239.

24. Bonvalot S, Miceli R, Berselli M, Causeret S, Colombo C, Mariani L, Bouzaiene H, Le Péchoux C, Casali PG, Le Cesne A, Fiore M, Gronchi A. Aggressive surgery in retroperitoneal soft tissue sarcoma carried out at high-volume centers is safe and is associated with improved local control. Ann Surg Oncol. 2010;17(6):1507–14.

25. Hollenbeck BK, Wei Y, Birkmeyer JD. Volume, process of care, and operative mortality for cystectomy for bladder cancer. Urology. 2007;69(5):871–5. https://doi.org/10.1016/j. urology.2007.01.040.

26. Keyes M, Crook J, Morris WJ, Morton G, Pickles T, Usmani N, Vigneault E. Canadian prostate brachytherapy in 2012. Can Urol Assoc J. 2013;7(1–2):51–8. https://doi.org/10.5489/cuaj.218.

27. Smith GD, Pickles T, Crook J, Martin AG, Vigneault E, Cury FL, et al. Brachytherapy improves biochemical failurefree survival in low- and intermediate-risk prostate cancer compared with

conventionally fractionated external beam radiation therapy: a propensity score matched analysis. Int J Radiat Oncol Biol Phys. 2015;91:505–16.

28. Wang Y, Sankreacha R, Al-Hebshi A, et al. Comparative study of dosimetry between high-dose-rate and permanent prostate implant brachytherapies in patients with prostate adenocarcinoma. Brachytherapy. 2006;5:251–5.

29. Morton G, Walker-Dilks C, Baldassarre F, et al. The delivery of brachytherapy for cervical cancer: organizational and technical advice to facilitate high-quality care in Ontario: guideline recommendations. Report Date: November 11, 2009.

30. Rosenblatt E. Planning national radiotherapy services. Front Oncol. 2014;4:315.

31. Page BR, Hudson AD, Brown DW, et al. Cobalt, linac, or other: what is the best solution for radiation therapy in developing countries. Int J Radiat Oncol Biol Phys. 2014;89:476–80.

32. Canadian Association for Accreditation of Ambulatory Surgery Facilities. Criteria for Accreditation of Ambulatory Surgical Facilities.

33. Australian and New Zealand College of Anaesthetists Recommendations for the Post-Anaesthesia Recovery Room.

34. Peeters A, Grutters JPC, Pijls-Johannesma M, et al. How costly is particle therapy? Cost analysis of external beam radiotherapy with carbon-ions, protons and photons. Radiother Oncol. 2010;95(1):45–53.

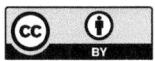

Chapter 7
Oncology Nursing Care

Jennifer Frith and Nelson J. Chao

Cancer is a leading cause of death worldwide, accounting for nearly 10 million deaths in 2020 [1]. This is due to many risk factors such as aging society, alcohol abuse, smoking, obesity, and lack of physical activity [2]. It is essential to deliver high-quality nursing care, from prevention and screening to end-of-life care. As research and scientific discoveries are incorporated into cancer treatment, nurses working in the oncology field should be well educated and be prepared to play an integral role in delivering complex treatment regimens and targeted cellular therapies. Therefore, focusing on specialized oncology nursing practice through advanced education will ensure successful care delivery.

By utilizing established standards and competencies to provide oncology nursing care, nurses will improve their knowledge and skill set. Nurses new to oncology, as well as experienced nurses from other specialties, should receive the required competencies to provide high-quality care to cancer patients. According to the Institute of Medicine [3], these include leadership, health policy, system improvement, research and evidence-based practice, teamwork and collaboration, community and public health, geriatrics, and oncology. Documentation supporting the development and validation of nursing competency is frequently required of accreditation agencies, including the American College of Surgeons and The Joint Commission, as part of the accreditation and reaccreditation process [4].

Any oncology setting should have policies to document any additional qualifications of specialized staff providing care to the cancer patient, especially regarding chemotherapy administration and documentation. The 2016 updated American

J. Frith (✉)
Inpatient Oncology and ABMT, Durham, NC, USA
e-mail: Jennifer.frith@duke.edu

N. J. Chao
Division of Hematologic Malignancies and Cellular Therapy/BMT, Global Cancer/Duke Cancer Institute/Duke Global Health Institute, Durham, NC, USA
e-mail: Nelson.chao@duke.edu

© The Author(s) 2022
M. Aljurf et al. (eds.), *The Comprehensive Cancer Center*,
https://doi.org/10.1007/978-3-030-82052-7_7

Society of Clinical Oncology/Oncology Nursing Society (ONS) chemotherapy administration safety standards recommend a minimum expectation for ordering, preparing, and administering chemotherapy [5]. There should be a comprehensive program for initial and ongoing oncology education requirements for all staff and a dedicated time frame for onboarding all new hires within the institution.

Oncology nursing continues to progress and can differ significantly across cultures. Currently, oncology nurses work in diverse settings such as hospitals, private physician clinics, outpatient infusions, radiation centers, home health agencies, and community settings, supporting many oncology disciplines. The oncology nurse's roles vary from a community focus of screening, detection, and prevention to a more intensive care focus such as blood and marrow transplantation. Regardless of the setting, nurses working in cancer care are responsible for focusing on patient assessment, management of symptoms, education, coordination, and supportive care.

According to the World Health Organization (WHO), there is a shortage of 7.2 million healthcare workers concerning health needs, whereas the report by the "Third Global Forum on Human Resources for Health" estimates that by 2035, the nursing deficit will reach 12.9 million [6]. With the growing shortages of health care professionals skilled in providing cancer care, the focus should be on providing oncology-specific training and competencies. Nursing staff shortages affect the quality or quantity of healthcare and decrease nurses' motivation regarding comprehensive care provision or care based on scientific principles [7]. This may lead to work overload, burnout, and increased nursing turnover. It is imperative to assess each clinical area's nursing unit structure and staffing needs and develop a nursing care model focused on evidence-based patient-centered care.

Oncology Inpatient Clinical Service Unit

Oncology nurses play a vital role in delivering high-quality care to patients hospitalized with a cancer diagnosis. The oncology care nurse needs to develop a collaborative relationship with the physician to deliver exceptional comprehensive patient care. Depending on the type of clinical service unit (CSU) being established or maintained, the nurse–patient ratio must be assessed initially and again over time. By benchmarking with other institutions, identifying an appropriate ratio and skill mix can be validated for the individual unit type. Because of the increased acuity and workload on an oncology inpatient unit, registered nurses (RN) are a critical component of the healthcare delivery model. However, due to the limited number of RNs in many countries around the world, it is suggested each institution assesses the individual characteristics of their nurses, their work environments, and their patient population [8] to ensure the appropriate skill mix has been identified. For example, the inpatient blood and marrow transplant unit would use a primary model with highly trained nurses and a lower nurse–patient ratio due to the complexity of care being delivered. In contrast, a medical oncology unit may have a higher nurse–patient ratio but utilize non-licensed personnel to assist with care. Based on the clinical unit's care and scope, one must consider what their staff may require to meet patient needs.

With the administration of antineoplastic agents occurring mostly on inpatient units, a global standard is recommended to ensure safe handling and administration for the care nurses by following the Oncology Nursing Society (ONS) guidelines. Nurses working in cancer care are responsible for education before start of treatment, safe drug handling; two-person independent verification of chemotherapy with the calculation of drug dosage based on body surface area, insertion of intravenous lines or accessing central venous devices; and continuous intense monitoring to identify early recognition of oncologic emergencies. Nurses specifically working in radiation oncology require an additional skill set. During basic nurse training, many nurses do not have the opportunity to participate in any radiation-related courses. To prevent nurses from exposure, it is necessary to provide the healthcare nurse with the appropriate knowledge of radioactive contamination. The nurse will also be responsible for symptom management assessment of skin rashes and communication of any toxicities identified.

Ambulatory Setting

Although an inpatient care delivery model can be transitioned to an ambulatory model easily, an assessment is imperative to understand the model's cost-effectiveness and efficiency while supporting high-quality care and positive patient outcomes. With the increased number of complex oncology patients transitioning to ambulatory care, highly skilled nurses' requirements are as crucial as in the inpatient setting. Choosing the correct nursing care delivery model will need to include patient-centered care while considering the increased complexity of nursing care requirements, monitoring quality metrics and patient outcomes, and implementing cost-containment measures such as drug costs. No standard staffing model or nurse-to-patient ratio exists for ambulatory infusion or chemotherapy treatment and radiation centers [9].

With this fast-paced setting, including the rapid turnover of patients, experienced nurses may be preferred. Ambulatory settings should consider many variables when creating a staffing model, for example, the physical location assessment: freestanding clinic versus attached to the hospital, types of service provided, hours of operation, patient population mix, and care needs. Acuity-based models should not be based solely on the patient's time in the treatment center and consider the complex care being administered. Implementing supportive protocols such as electrolytes, blood supplementation, and fever workups allow nurses' autonomy and immediate care delivery with minimal delay.

Oncology Role Outside of the Clinical Setting

With cancer care transitioning to the ambulatory setting, patients and caregivers have to manage symptoms and side effects of treatment in their home. Many of these patients travel from afar to receive cancer therapy. The nurse should serve as the first line of communication. From the referral process to end-of-life care, the patient and or/family should be able to contact an oncology nurse by phone during their entire continuum of care. By developing a triage support system, the patient will have consistent communication with their health care team, allow for emotional support, and identify any emergencies. A nursing care triage model can support various settings, including ambulatory clinics and outpatient infusion areas, supporting increased patient satisfaction and positive patient outcomes. For example, for a patient calling with a fever, an evidence-based protocol with a physician order set embedded would reduce the time to receive antibiotics and potentially decrease a patient's length of stay in the hospital. It is also essential to assess hours of operation and a need for 24-hour access.

With global technology increasing and patients traveling from afar, is there an opportunity, when able, to leverage telehealth for remote symptom management. For some remote geographic areas, telecommunication technology may allow nurses a vehicle to provide nursing care to patients in alternative care sites such as patient homes, shelters, and nursing homes. Nurses can provide numerous services in these areas, such as patient education, coordination of care, arranging appointments, and symptom management with physician resource support. Utilizing telehealth and other types of remote technology, nursing can help eliminate barriers, time, and distance a patient may experience living in remote areas and assess as part of the care delivery model.

Survivorship/Palliative Care and Hospice

As cancer survivors grow, nurses often play a pivotal role during the survivorship plan of care. Once a patient's treatment regimen is completed, patients are often at a loss of managing their long-term side effects, emotional distress, and economic burden lacking the knowledge they can reach out to address these concerns. By providing specialized training for long-term oncology care, nurses can deliver guidance, education, and appropriate referrals to address various issues. These real-life situations can help the cancer care community develop optimal care algorithms and identify the interprofessional team members for survivorship care delivery [10]. Depending on how far the patient may travel for cancer survivorship care, a telehealth platform may benefit a particular institution.

Palliative care is necessary to support comprehensive cancer care. As the trend in healthcare moves from a fee-for-service model to a patient-centered, value-based model, the expectation is that an increase will occur in the integration of palliative care into comprehensive oncology care [11]. Nurses have learned to incorporate caregiver goals into the plan of care. A cancer diagnosis often results in distress in the physical, psychosocial, spiritual, and emotional domains of care. Today, palliative care nursing focuses on care delivery to individual patients and families, within specific disease populations, and palliative care issues within health care and society as a whole entity. Proper training is essential to have the knowledge and skillset to address the numerous facets of cancer. The Hospice and Palliative Nursing Certification (CHPN) was developed in 1994 to support additional education and guidance in this field of nursing. Once the care nurse has a few years of experience, certification is recommended to support continued education in this field.

With the increased aging population in developed countries worldwide, patients may choose to have end-of-life care in various settings such as a hospital, outpatient facilities, or at home. Both new and seasoned oncology nurses need to be comfortable providing end-of-life nursing care. Training programs exist, End-of-Life Nursing Education Consortium (ELNEC), focusing on nursing education to deliver optimal end-of-life care to patients and their families [12]. Burnout is a significant concern for the oncology nurse delivering end-of-life care. To support resilience and sustain the workforce, oncology nurses need strategies on how to support these complex patients, their families, and themselves to be successful in delivering high-quality end-of-life care.

In conclusion, the care nurse plays a vital role in delivering oncology care, including administering multiple and complex treatment regimens. The coordination encompasses direct patient care, documentation in the medical record, participation in therapy, symptom management, organization of referrals to other healthcare providers, family and patient education, and diagnosis, therapy, and follow-up. Providing continuous education and competencies to the care nurse, implementing evidence-based practice, and identifying the appropriate nursing care delivery model will support quality care delivery in these complex environments.

References

1. Ferlay J, Ervik M, Lam F, Colombet M, Mery L, Piñeros M, et al. Global Cancer Observatory: Cancer Today. Lyon: International Agency for Research on Cancer; 2020 (https://gco.iarc.fr/today).
2. Torre LA, Bray F, Siegel RL, Ferlay J, Lortet-Tieulent J, Jemal A. Global cancer statistics, 2012. CA Cancer J Clin. 2015;65(2):87–108.
3. Institute of Medicine. The future of nursing: leading change, advancing health. Washington, DC: National Academies Press; 2011. https://doi.org/10.17226/12956.
4. Gaguski ME, George K, Bruce SD, Brucker E, Leija C, LeFebvre KB, Mackey H. Oncology nurse generalist competencies: oncology nursing society's initiative to establish best practice. Clin J Oncolo Nurs. 2017;21(6):679–87. https://doi.org/10.1188/17.CJON.679-687
5. Oncology Nursing Society. Oncology nurse generalist competencies. 2016. Retrieved from http://bit.ly/2fisCmx.
6. Marć M, Bartosiewicz A, Burzyńska J, Chmiel Z, Januszewicz P. A nursing shortage–a prospect of global and local policies. Int Nurs Rev. 2019;66(1):9–16.

7. Dehghan-Nayeri N, Shali M, Navabi N, Ghaffari F. Perspectives of oncology unit nurse manag-ers on missed nursing care: a qualitative study. Asia-Pacific J Oncol Nurs. 2018;5(3):327–36. https://doi.org/10.4103/apjon.apjon_6_18.
8. Kouatly IA, Nassar N, Nizam M, Badr LK. Evidence on nurse staffing ratios and patient out-comes in a low-income country: implications for future research and practice. Worldviews Evid-Based Nurs. 2018;15(5):353–60. https://doi.org/10.1111/wvn.12316
9. Society, O. ONS staffing position statement: ambulatory treatment centers. Oncol Nurs Forum. 2020;47(1):15.
10. Rosenzweig MQ, Kota K, van Londen G. Interprofessional management of cancer survivor-ship: new models of care. Semin Oncol Nurs. 2017;33(4):449–58. WB Saunders
11. Dailey E. The evidence behind integrating palliative care into oncology practice. Clin J Oncol Nurs. 2016;20(4):368.
12. Glover TL, Garvan C, Nealis RM, Citty SW, Derrico DJ. Improving end-of- life care knowledge among senior baccalaureate nursing students. Am J Hospice Palliat Med®. 2017;34(10):938–45.

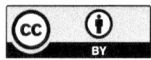

Chapter 8
Laboratory/Pathology Services and Blood Bank

Kathryn M. Fleming, Matthias Klammer, and Mickey B. C. Koh

Comprehensive cancer care (CCC) brings together clinical services, research and education for the benefit of cancer patients. The main input of laboratories and pathology services to CCC service is rapid access to high-quality diagnostics, which will be much of the focus of this chapter. In addition, the support of laboratories toward education, research and development is also essential to attain the status of world-class CCC, and this is reflected in the definition given by the National Cancer Institute [1].

Pivotal to all high-quality cancer care is the ability to achieve accurate and detailed diagnosis so as to enable prognostication and treatment strategies. This has increasingly moved from morphological and descriptive diagnostic techniques to a molecular landscape where tumour genomes are interrogated for their tumour signatures. All of this sits within the purview of pathology and its laboratories.

The other essential role played by the laboratory/pathology services is the support of patients undergoing treatment and follow-up: delivery of safe blood, a stem cell processing lab, rapid analysis of blood samples, identification of infectious agents amongst a host of other functions.

World-leading CCC centres are not only international reference centres for patient care, their genomics research and access to large volume clinical material and data aim to embed personalised medicine as part of patient care, likely in investigational clinical trials [2–4]. The ability of laboratory and pathology services to

K. M. Fleming (✉) · M. Klammer
Department of Haematology, St Georges University Hospital, London, UK

M. B. C. Koh
Department of Haematology, St George's University Hospital, London, UK

Stem Cell Transplantation, Institute of Infection and Immunity, St George's Medical School, University of London, London, UK

Cell Therapy Facility, Health Sciences Authority, Singapore, Singapore

© The Author(s) 2022
M. Aljurf et al. (eds.), *The Comprehensive Cancer Center*,
https://doi.org/10.1007/978-3-030-82052-7_8

63

obtain, analyse and integrate ever-increasing amounts of complex information helps the modern cancer multidisciplinary team (MDT) to achieve this goal.

We have subdivided this chapter into the broad headings of what we consider to be the fundamental roles of pathology and laboratory service in the CCC as follows:

1. Laboratory and pathology support for screening programs and arriving at a cancer diagnosis
2. Laboratory and pathology support for maintaining quality supportive care throughout cancer treatment
3. Specific pathology support for running stem cell transplant/cellular therapy programs and pathology support for running cancer clinical trials and research.

Relevant to all aspects of laboratory and pathology services in CCC is the requirement for *accreditation* or *external review* and control. Accreditation is public recognition by a healthcare body of the achievement of standards by a healthcare organization, demonstrated through an independent external peer assessment of that organization's level of performance in relation to the standards. Accreditation standards may be regional or national, or they may be international and aim to define quality standards and achieve uniformity in a health system [5]. Whatever laboratory or pathology service you provide, this process is being used worldwide to ensure that results from labs are comparable, clinically useful and safe.

A CCC centre would be expected to drive the development of local, national or international evidence-based guidelines in an area of cancer care. The ability of a CCC centre's laboratory and pathology service to access high-quality data, with high throughput of patient cases and samples would be best suited to this function. This is reflected in major world CCC centres' laboratory involvement in national and international guidelines seen today, for example,

- Comprehensive Cancer Center Ulm, Ulm, Germany – input into European Society of Medical Oncology (ESMO) guidelines in chronic myeloid leukaemia, chronic lymphocytic leukaemia and acute myeloid leukaemia [6–8].
- INCLIVA, University of Valencia, Spain – input into several ESMO guidelines including metastatic colorectal cancer, anal cancer, hereditary GI cancers, hepatocellular cancer [9–12].
- Dana-Farber Cancer Institute, Boston, MA, US – into ESMO guidelines for advanced breast cancer, but also many American Society of Clinical Oncology guidelines [13, 14].

Information management, maintaining of databases and storage of laboratory/ pathology data, as well as management of laboratory research data are also major considerations but will be not covered in this chapter. Most CCC centres have invested heavily and developed systems capable of dealing with vast data quantities.

Laboratory and Pathology Support for Screening Programs and Arriving at a Cancer Diagnosis

The input of laboratory/pathology services into the modern cancer MDT or "tumour board" contributes to the formation of a full "integrated" cancer diagnostic report. An integrated report at its most basic, from a lab/path perspective, needs cellular pathology and histopathology. However, CCC centres add immunohistochemistry, cytogenetics, molecular, genomic analysis and immunophenotyping (particularly in haemato-oncology) as key components of the integrated report, given that many diagnoses will not be complete or therapeutic options will not be fully explored without these techniques [15].

An MDT or "tumour board" will need to integrate all of the above information with clinical and radiological data, and it is in part the responsibility of laboratory and pathology services to achieve this. It is crucially this "integration" process that is the hallmark of CCC, and then "translating" the integrated report into excellent care and facilitating patient-centred research. Support and personal attendance of senior scientists, laboratory staff and pathologists is increasingly vital to the modern cancer MDT.

In addition to individual patient care, population-based cancer screening programs that may be linked to CCC centres will also depend on laboratory and pathology support from cervical pap smear cytology to faecal occult testing to supporting research-based programs like UK-based 100,000 Genomes Project [16].

Cellular pathology and histopathology will require the capability for specimen fixation, embedding into paraffin, tissue slicing, and staining. The pathologists reporting of samples at CCC centres will frequently require subspecialty expertise or access to such expertise via international networks, especially for rare cancers. In many cases, this is facilitated by telepathology which may include sharing of selected static images, whole-slide scanning, dynamic non-robotic telemicroscopy, and dynamic robotic tele-microscopy. Selected static image sharing can be as simple as a microscope, digital camera, and Internet connection and has been successfully used in Butaro Cancer Center of Excellence in Rwanda, where a static-image telepathology system was established after a training period for field selection, in collaboration with the Dana-Farber/Brigham and Women's Cancer Center [17, 18].

Immunohistochemistry (IHC) now provides important diagnostic and prognostic information as well as guiding therapeutic options for cancer care. IHC, the application of antibody stains with a chromogenic or fluorescent readout to identify tumour markers, their quantity and location and interpretation of significance is nowadays ubiquitous. An important choice to be made is whether to carry out IHC on formalin-fixed, paraffin-embedded samples or on fresh frozen samples. Paraffin embedding offers superior tissue/cell morphology, but antigenicity is potentially compromised by the fixation required for paraffin-embedded samples. A CCC would require access to facilities capable of freezing samples, storing samples and access to many antibody panels that often need refrigerated storage themselves [19, 20].

Cytogenetic studies, the study of chromosomal structure, or karyotyping was first utilised in cancer diagnostics in the 1960s with the discovery of the Philadelphia chromosome. Classical karyotyping or banding techniques (G-, Q-, R- banding) nowadays is a limited, but useful genome-wide screening tool. However, it requires a high mitotic index of cells, good chromosomal morphology and is time-consuming. The drive for rapid results and the ability to analyse preserved samples in interphase has pushed molecular cytogenetic techniques such as fluorescence in situ hybridisation (FISH), multicolour-FISH (M-FISH and SKY) and competitive genome hybridization (CGH) into the forefront of modern cancer diagnostics. The ability of the CCC centre to bridge basic research to clinical practice using these techniques has expanded rapidly in recent years. Access to reliable and specific marker probes and increasingly automated methods would help to facilitate expansion of testing capabilities in what has traditionally been a highly labour-intensive technique.

Molecular cytogenetic analysis is particularly useful in haematological and soft tissue tumours albeit historically less used in solid tumours due to a scarcity of specific associated cytogenetic abnormalities and difficulty in processing the sample for analysis. As more and more targetable tumour markers are identified, FISH studies are increasingly useful to identify upfront whether patients can be offered targeted treatment. Some examples of solid tumour FISH use are: differential diagnosis between teratoid/rhabdoid and medulloblastoma/primitive neuroectodermal tumours and dual colour FISH for HER-2 in breast cancer as a prognostic marker and predictor or therapy response [21].

Genetic analysis of tumour and patient DNA in modern cancer care has been revolutionized with the recent advances of next-generation sequencing (NGS), hybridization capture targeted multigene panels and computational data analysis [22]. Discussing the various genome analysis techniques, their implementation and practical aspects are beyond the scope of this chapter; however, there are important principles to consider. Technical challenges related to the quantity and quality of tumour sample will have a direct impact on your ability to use genetic studies related to your laboratory's knowledge and equipment. Sample preparation methodologies are crucial to maximising the chance of obtaining useful information from what may be a small, poor quality and formalin-fixed biopsy sample.

Most centres now run tumour-specific multi-gene panels which are "trade-off" between slow turnaround, labour-intensive genome-wide screening approaches and potentially low-yield single mutation screening with Sanger sequencing. A myeloid gene panel for suspected Acute Myeloid Leukaemia, for example, could contain >20 genes which are of high specificity and sensitivity for the disease and may directly alter prognosis and treatment options, for example, IDH mutations [23]. The decision as to the depth, breadth and methodology used in multi-gene panels will be very much centre-dependent, taking into consideration the throughput, turn-around time, equipment, cost and skill set of your centre. Hereditary cancer syndromes are a field of CCC that has greatly benefited from massively parallel sequencing, as most known familial cancer syndromes are represented by several distinct genes that may cause similar clinical manifestation. The ability to scrutinize many known or potential disease-causing mutations is very powerful [22]. For instance, in Lynch syndrome or Hereditary non-polyposis colorectal cancer – a screen might involve NGS to identify MLH1, MSH2, MSH6, PMS2, or EPCAM mutations, then PCR-based microsatellite instability testing [24].

The post-genomic era has created vast quantities of data for CCC, which in most centres has spawned a "cancer genomics MDT", a genomics review board (as in the UK) or "molecular tumour board" (as in US institutions like Brigham and Women's Hospital) [25, 26]. The genetic complexity of cancer, the relevance of mutational changes and the application of multiple NGS-based assays create a challenge in the interpretation and clinical application of this data. Increasingly, this makes it necessary for pathologists and molecular scientists to be core and essential members of the multidisciplinary team in deliberating the final clinical recommendation based on multiple complex test results [27, 28].

Other molecular studies for diagnosis and disease monitoring, such as tumour markers, immunological studies such as protein electrophoresis and high-performance liquid chromatography (HPLC) are discussed in the section "Laboratory and Pathology support for maintaining quality supportive cancer care".

Immunophenotyping using flow cytometry (FCM) is extensively used in haemato-oncology but can also be ancillary to the diagnosis of metastatic adenocarcinoma and malignant mesothelioma in effusions. The limitations in haematological cell morphological analysis are vastly compensated for by this technique; it can be performed in a matter of hours and provides key information for the diagnosis, classification and monitoring of many haematological malignancies. Single-cell suspensions of solid tumours and circulating tumour cells are being used and are likely to be of increasing clinical use as more research is developed. Panels of FCM markers are also used in the assessment of neuroblastomas, primitive neuroectodermal tumours, Wilms' tumour, rhabdomyosarcomas and germ cell tumours [29]. FCM can not only provide analytic data, but also be used as a cell sorting method to enrich cell populations for genetic studies. With the use of multi-colour FCM, laboratory scientists and clinicians will both need to have an understanding of the diagnostic relevance and interpretation of results. It is of key importance that clinician and scientist are sharing information.

It is also important to mention that, although we have discussed cytogenetic, genetic and immunophenotypic analyses in the "diagnosis" section, all are of immense value in disease monitoring and monitoring of treatment response. With the concept of minimal/measurable residual disease (MRD) and the emerging knowledge that tumour genetic evolution can influence relapse and treatment failure risk, there is an increasing challenge to pathologists, geneticists and laboratory services to standardise procedures, increase testing capacity and engage with clinicians throughout the patient's treatment.

Laboratory and Pathology Support for Maintaining Quality Supportive Cancer Care

Microbiological services are essential in a CCC centre, as immunocompromised patients undergoing chemotherapy/immunotherapy often are highly vulnerable to infection. This includes suspected infections that may be rare or atypical, antimicrobial resistance monitoring, monitoring of therapeutic drug levels (e.g. gentamicin, vancomycin, voriconazole, ganciclovir) and translating microbiological research results into practice in cancer patients.

Prevention of infectious disease, such as screening of blood-borne virus exposure prior to chemotherapy, will require serological study facilities, screening for Healthcare Associated Infections (HAI) potential, for example, MSRA and swabbing may also be required in large healthcare facilities. The treatment of infectious disease during chemotherapy will require the capability for blood and fluid bacterial and mycological culture, viral PCR capabilities (e.g. respiratory virus swab PCR) and senior microbiology input to interpret results and advise on therapy options.

Biochemistry and haematology laboratory services with capabilities specific to cancer care are vital in CCC. Coagulation studies, automated cell counting technology and manual differential cell counting in blood and marrow samples, provided in haematology laboratory services are both diagnostic in their own capacity (for haematological malignancy and bone marrow infiltration of other solid tumours) as well as supportive for all aspects of CCC. They allow monitoring myelosuppression during chemotherapy/radiotherapy, monitoring response to infectious disease, determining safety for cancer-related procedures (e.g. coagulation assays prior to surgical resection), as well as the facility to deal with complex problems of haemostasis in cancer patients (e.g. complex venous thrombo-embolism, anti-Xa monitoring, acquired haemophilia, etc).

Biochemistry support for CCC at its core entails electrolyte monitoring, surrogates for organ function or damage, for example, U&E, LFTs, BNP, protein-based and immunological assays for disease monitoring used in solid and liquid tumours, for example, prostate-specific antigen (PSA), cancer antigen 125 (CA-125), carcinoembryonic antigen (CEA) and serum protein electrophoresis, serum free light chain analysis and HPLC (the latter specifically for diagnosis of phaeochromocytoma, neuroblastoma and carcinoid syndrome) [30, 31].

Blood bank and transfusion support: This includes the acquisition, storage and appropriate use of blood products. The laboratory infrastructure required for the storage of blood products and the information technology support used in electronic cross-matching, product storage tracking and monitoring fridge performance is considerable, but necessary in large cancer centres particularly in those specializing in haemato-oncology. Laboratory support needs to be provided to clinicians to guide the appropriate use of blood products and to provide appropriate protocols for emergency situations, such as massive haemorrhage. Laboratory support is required for the detection of complex auto-, allo- and drug-induced antibody presentations in the multiply transfused or treated patient (e.g. Daratumumab) and management/

investigation of transfusion reactions or product refractoriness. Access to irradiated blood products is crucial for many cancer patients for prevention of transfusion-associated Graft vs Host Disease as well as access to HLA/HPA-matched products in platelet refractory cases.

Pathology Support for Running Stem Cell Transplant/ Cellular Therapies

Haematopoietic stem cell transplantation (HSCT) and cellular therapies (CAR-T) require many unique laboratory facilities. Broadly, we have subdivided these into:

1. Biochemistry, microbiology and histopathology services
2. Histocompatibility and immunogenetics (H&I)
3. Apheresis and cell management
4. Chimerism studies

1. Monitoring of drug levels specific to stem cell transplantation monitoring such as ciclosporin and tacrolimus. Due to the highly immunosuppressive nature of stem cell transplantation, more intensive microbiological screening and monitoring is required, such as regular CMV, EBV, and adenovirus viraemia screening (preferably by PCR testing), pre-transplant serology HIV, HTLV, viral hepatitis, syphilis, toxoplasmosis and other mandatory tests for communicable diseases. Histopathologists with expertise in identifying graft-versus-host disease (GvHD) from biopsy samples are required to support a haematopoietic stem cell transplant service. HSCT and CAR-T centres must have a 24-hour on-site blood bank, haematology and biochemistry laboratory services and access to stem cell collection and processing facilities.
2. Apheresis is the most commonly used technique for stem cell collection requiring staff with both clinical and laboratory training in the use of this procedure. CCCs will need access to facilities for storage and cryopreservation of haematopoietic cells from a variety of sources. Close coordination with apheresis units is required to ensure adequate CD34+ cell doses from stem cell collections. Furthermore, HSCT centres require the preparation of T cell therapeutic (TC-T) aliquots (formerly called donor lymphocytes infusions or DLI) in measured CD3 doses. Quality assurance methodologies by validated procedures will be necessary such as the use of microbiological tests to assure the suitability of donors and the safety of products. The use of flow-cytometric and/or tissue culture assay systems to demonstrate progenitor viability and process suitability is mandatory [32–34].
3. Histocompatibility & Immunogenetics (H&I) services in support of cancer care are mostly involved with HLA typing and antibody screening which is mandatory for all allogeneic transplant centres. However, H&I is also important for other ancillary services with respect to cancer such as screening for

heparin-induced thrombocytopenia, HLA-polymorphism testing (for lapatinib-induced DILI in breast cancer) and the diagnosis of platelets refractoriness (using PIFT and MAIPA studies). In recent years, accredited H&I laboratory facilities perform timely DNA-based intermediate and high-resolution HLA typing via a form of sequence specific priming, or NGS. The H&I lab will allow clinician access to bone marrow registries to facilitate access to matched unrelated donors and cord blood registries [32, 35].

4. Recent advances and understanding in cellular immunotherapy as a major therapeutic pillar in cancer treatment, especially, haemato-oncology has increased the reliance on and interdependency of the stem cell processing laboratory and more advanced Good Manufacturing Practices (cGMP) cell therapy facilities, often under the management of pathology. This will require expert staff individuals trained in the manufacture of complex cell therapy therapeutic products [35]. The area of chimeric antigen receptor T-cell therapy (CAR-T) is an example of this with numerous worldwide clinical trials and with the cell therapy laboratory requiring access to apheresis, bespoke CAR-T manufacture requiring viral vectors, genetic modification, packaging, systems for T cell expansion and vapour liquid phase nitrogen storage [44].

Pathology Support for Running Cancer Clinical Trials and Research

Laboratories and pathology services are integral to the running of clinical trials and biomedical cancer research. Development and discovery of genetic/biomarkers of disease (or disease classification and prognostic stratification), drug development, nanotechnology, cellular therapy development, gene therapy are a few broad examples. Education and training of academics, clinicians and laboratory staff is at the forefront of comprehensive cancer care, and this includes both standard-of-care clinical practice and investigational clinical trials supported by ethical guidance at national and international level (e.g. FDA Good Laboratory practice (US), EU clinical trials, Good Clinical Practice, the Declaration of Helsinki and the Human Tissue Act (UK)) [36].

From a laboratory perspective, apart from the above-mentioned facilities (high-quality diagnostic techniques, monitoring of biochemistry and haematology lab support), clinical drug trials may need the facilities to synthesize and purify new compounds, assess drug pharmacokinetics and pharmacodynamics in cell, animal or human subject samples. Laboratory involvement can be from drug discovery and development right through to post-market safety monitoring.

Biobanks, with respect to cancer care, are the storage of large numbers of biological samples for use in research – ranging from tumour tissue samples, genetic material and drug levels or biomarkers from serum, saliva, stool, etc. Biobanks are often utilized by major CCC research centres, giving research teams rapid access to vast quantities of samples spanning a long time period [37–40]. Although biobanks are often disease-oriented, for example lung cancer, they may be population-based to determine susceptibility of disease development.

Laboratory support in biobanking will require secure, well-maintained, long-term cryogenic storage facilities (with temperature control documentation and backup systems in case of power failure), and sample tracking capabilities. Traceability is critical and the strict adherence to protocols ensuring appropriate patient informed consent. Standard operating procedures for laboratory sample handling and processing are also highly desirable for reproducibility and data reliability. Such biobanking facilities are often required to comply with stringent operating policies and meticulous laboratory support in order to gain a human tissue act license [41]. To this end, many international groups have written "best practice guidelines" for example, International Society for Biological and Environmental Repositories (ISBER) and NCI Best Practices for Biospecimen Resources. They have also tried to address the ethical concerns that often surround biobanks such as ownership of specimens and the extent as to which specimen donor can consent to all forms of future research [42, 43].

In conclusion, pathology and its laboratories are central in supporting every facet of cancer care in a CCC center, from diagnosis, biobanking, patient support during treatment, research, therapeutic drug manufacture and development. The ability to support all of this will always need to be balanced against time and costs. As such, any strategic planning for the setting up of a CCC center should allow for careful deliberation and meticulous planning on the scope and breadth of pathology services to be set up.

References

1. NIH, National cancer institute, US department of health and human science. URL last accessed 4/10/20: https://www.cancer.gov/publications/dictionaries/cancer-terms/def/comprehensive-cancer-center.
2. Stanley Kimmel, Johns Hopkins medicine. URL last accessed 4/10/20: https://www.hopkinsmedicine.org/kimmel_cancer_center/our_approach.html.
3. Memorial Sloan Kettering, NY, US. URL last accessed 4/10/20: https://www.mskcc.org/.
4. MD Anderson, Texas, US. URL last accessed 4/10/20: https://www.mdanderson.org/.
5. Gospodarowicz M, Trypuc J, D'Cruz A, et al. Cancer Services and the Comprehensive Cancer Center. In: Gelband H, Jha P, Sankaranarayanan R, et al., editors. Cancer: disease control priorities, vol. 3. 3rd ed. Washington (DC): The International Bank for Reconstruction and Development / The World Bank; 2015. Chapter 11. Available from: URL last accessed 4/10/20: https://www.ncbi.nlm.nih.gov/books/NBK343637/.
6. Hochhaus A, Saussele S, Rosti G, et al. Chronic myeloid leukaemia: ESMO clinical practice guidelines. Ann Oncol. 2017;28 (suppl 4):iv41–iv51.
7. Eichhorst B, Robak T, Montserrat E, Ghia P, Hillmen P, Hallek M, Buske C. Chronic lymphocytic leukaemia: ESMO clinical practice guidelines. Ann Oncol. 2015;26(suppl 5):v78–84.

8. Heuser M, Ofran Y, Boissel N, Brunet S, Mauri C, et al. Clinical practice guidelines – acute myeloid leukaemia in adult patients. Ann Oncol. 2020;31(0):0–0.
9. Cutsem V, Cervantes A, Adam R, Sobrero A, et al. ESMO Consensus Guidelines for the Management of Patients with Metastatic Colorectal Cancer first published online: July 5, 2016E.
10. Glynne-Jones R, Nilsson PJ, Aschele C, Goh V, et al. Anal Cancer: ESMO-ESSO-ESTRO clinical practice guidelines. Published in 2014. Ann Oncol. 2014;25 (suppl 3):iii10–iii20.
11. Stjepanovic N, Moreira L, Carneiro F, Balaguer F, Cervantes A, Balmaña J. Martinelli E on behalf of the ESMO Guidelines Committee. Hereditary gastrointestinal cancers: ESMO clinical practice guidelines for diagnosis, treatment and follow-up. Ann Oncol. 2019;00:1–34.
12. Vogel A, Cervantes A, Chau I, Daniele B, Llovet J, et al. on behalf of the ESMO Guidelines Committee. Hepatocellular carcinoma: ESMO clinical practice guidelines for diagnosis, treatment and follow-up. Ann Oncol. 2018;29 (Suppl 4):iv238–iv255.
13. Cardoso F, Senkus E, Costa A, Papadopoulos E, et al. Consensus recommendations – Advanced Breast Cancer (ABC 4) 4th ESO–ESMO International Consensus Guidelines for Advanced Breast Cancer (ABC 4) published in 2018. Ann Oncol. 2018;29:1634–57.
14. Hassett MJ, Somerfield M, Baker ER. Management of Male Breast Cancer: ASCO guideline. J Clin Oncol. 2020;38(16):1849–63. https://doi.org/10.1200/JCO.19.03120.
15. Haematological cancers. Quality standard [QS150]. National Institute of Clinical Excellence (NICE). Published date: 01 June 2017. URL last accessed: 4/10/20 https://www.nice.org.uk/guidance/qs150/chapter/Quality-statement-1-Integrated-reporting.
16. The National Genomics Research and Healthcare Knowledgebase v5, Genomics England. doi:https://doi.org/10.6084/m9.figshare.4530893.v5. 2019. URL last accessed 4/10/20: https://www.genomicsengland.co.uk/about-genomics-england/the-100000-genomes-project/cancer/.
17. Mpunga T, Hedt-Gauthier BL, Tapela N, Nshimiyimana I, Muvugabigwi G, et al. Implementation and validation of telepathology triage at cancer Referral Center in Rural Rwanda. Jr. J Glob Oncol. 2016;2(2):76–82.
18. Pantanowitz LJ. Digital images and the future of digital pathology. Pathol Inform. 2010;1
19. Crosby K, Simendinger J, Grange C, Ferrante M, Bernier T, Standen C. Immunohistochemistry protocol for paraffin-embedded tissue sections. JoVE J. 2014; https://doi.org/10.3791/5064. URL last accessed 4/10/20: https://www.jove.com/video/5064/immunohistochemistry-protocol-for-paraffin-embedded-tissue-sections.
20. Gralow JR, Krakauer E, Anderson BO, Ilbawi A, Porter P, et al. Core elements for provision of cancer care and control in low and middle income countries. In: Knaul FM, Gralow J, Atun R, Bhadelia A, for the Global Task Force on Expanded Access to Cancer Care and Control in Developing Countries, editors. Closing the cancer divide: an equity imperative. Boston: Harvard Global Equity Initiative; 2012. p. 125–65.
21. Varella-Garcia M. Molecular cytogenetics in solid tumors: laboratorial tool for diagnosis. Progn Ther. 2003;8(1):45–58. https://doi.org/10.1634/theoncologist.8-1-45.
22. Sokolenko AP, Imyanitov EN. Molecular diagnostics in clinical oncology. Front Mol Biosci. 2018;5:76. https://doi.org/10.3389/fmolb.2018.00076.
23. Peter MacCallum Cancer centre. Victoria, Australia. Request form in suspected haematological malignancies. URL last accessed 4/10/20: https://www.petermac.org/sites/default/files/page/downloads/Molecular%20Haematology%20Request%20Slip%2004.05.18.pdf.
24. Mayo clinic. Lynch Syndrome Panel, Varies. URL last accessed 4/10/20: https://www.mayo-cliniclabs.com/test-catalog/Overview/64333.
25. Titus K. College of American Pathologists. CAP today. From tumor board, an integrated diagnostic report, 2014 URL last accessed 4/10/20: https://www.captodayonline.com/tumor-board-integrated-diagnostic-report/.

26. Moore DA, Kushnir M, Mak G. Prospective analysis of 895 patients on a UK genomics review board. ESMO Open. 2019;4(2):e000469. https://doi.org/10.1136/esmoopen-2018-000469. PMID: 31245058.
27. Berger MF, Mardis ER. The emerging clinical relevance of genomics in cancer medicine. Nat Rev Clin Oncol. 2018;15(6):353–65. https://doi.org/10.1038/s41571-018-0002-6.
28. Knepper TC, Bell GC, Hicks JK, et al. Key lessons learned from Moffitt's Molecular Tumor Board: the Clinical Genomics Action Committee experience. Oncologist. 2017;22(2):144–51. https://doi.org/10.1634/theoncologist.2016-0195. Epub 2017 Feb 8.
29. Pillai V, Dorfman DM. Flow cytometry of nonhematopoietic neoplasms. Acta Cytol. 2016;60(4):336–43. https://doi.org/10.1159/000448371. Epub 2016 Aug 27.
30. Peaston RT, Weinkove C. Measurement of catecholamines and their metabolites. Ann Clin Biochem. 2004;41(1):17–38.
31. Lionetto L, Lostia AM, Stigliano A, Cardelli P, Simmaco M. HPLC-mass spectrometry method for quantitative detection of neuroendocrine tumor markers: Vanillylmandelic acid, homovanillic acid and 5-hydroxyindoleacetic acid. Clin Chim Acta. PMID: 18760269. 2008, https://doi.org/10.1016/j.cca.2008.08.003.
32. National Health Service Blood and Transplant (UK). NHSBT. Processing and cryopreservation of stem cells. URL last accessed 4/10/20: https://hospital.blood.co.uk/patient-services/stem-cells/processing-and-cryopreservation-of-stem-cells/.
33. Rasheed W, Niederwieser DW, Aljurf M. Ch4. The HSCT Unit. In: The EBMT handbook: hematopoietic stem cell transplantation and cellular therapies [Internet]. 7th ed; 2019. URL last accessed 4/10/20: https://www.ncbi.nlm.nih.gov/books/NBK553974/.
34. Leemhuis T, Padley D, Keever-Taylor C, Niederwieser D, Teshima T, Lanza F, Chabannon C, Szabolcs P, Bazarbachi A, Koh MBC, Graft Processing Subcommittee of the Worldwide Network for Blood and Bone Marrow Transplantation (WBMT). Essential requirements for setting up a stem cell processing laboratory. Bone Marrow Transplant. 2014;49(8):1098–105. https://doi.org/10.1038/bmt.2014.104. Epub 2014 Jun 16.
35. National Health Service Blood and Transplant (UK). Information document 136/7. NHSBT Effective: 27/3/2020. URL last accessed 4/10/20: https://nhsbtdbe.blob.core.windows.net/umbraco-assets-corp/18149/inf136.pdf.
36. World Medical Association. Declaration of Helsinki: ethical principles for medical research involving human subjects. JAMA. 2013;310(20):2191–4. https://doi.org/10.1001/jama.2013.281053.
37. Grizzle WE, Bell WC, Sexton KC. Issues in collecting, processing and storing human tissues and associated information to support biomedical research. Cancer Biomark. 2010;9(1–6):531–49. https://doi.org/10.3233/CBM-2011-0183.
38. Patil S, Majumdar B, Awan KH, Gargi S, Sarode GS, Sarode SC, Gadbail AR, Gondivkar S. Cancer oriented biobanks: a comprehensive review. Oncol Rev. 2018;12(1):357. https://doi.org/10.4081/oncol.2018.357.
39. Paskal W, Paskal AM, Dębski T, Gryziak M, Jaworowski J. Aspects of modern biobank activity – comprehensive review. Pathol Oncol Res. 2018;24(4):771–85. https://doi.org/10.1007/s12253-018-0418-4.
40. Macleod AK, Liewald DC, McGilchrist MM, Morris AD, et al. Some principles and practices of genetic biobanking studies. Euro Resp J. 2009;33(2):419–25. https://doi.org/10.1183/09031936.00043508.
41. Human Tissue Act 2004 c.30, UK Public General Acts. URL last accessed 4/10/20: https://www.legislation.gov.uk/ukpga/2004/30/contents.

42. International Society for Biological and Environmental Repositories. Best Practices for Repositories: Collection, Storage, Retrieval and Distribution of Biological Materials for Research. 2012. URL last accessed 4/10/20: https://www.isber.org/page/BPR.
43. NCI Best Practices for Biospecimen Resources, 3rd ed. 2016. URL last accessed 4/10/20: https://cdn.ymaws.com/www.isber.org/resource/resmgr/Files/ISBER_Best_Practices_3rd_Edi.pdf.
44. Koh MB, Suck G. Cell therapy: promise fulfilled. Biologicals. 2012;40(3):214–7.

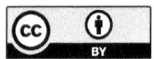

Chapter 9
Pharmacy Requirements for a Comprehensive Cancer Center

Lita Chew and Miko Chui Mei Thum

Introduction

Healthcare is experiencing significant challenges in recent years. The aging population and increasing prevalence of chronic diseases have led to increase in demand and complexity of medication regimens requiring major changes in the way cancer care is delivered. In addition, care providers face a consumer and patient base that is better informed and educated, technologically savvier with ready access to information through social networking and the Internet of things. Compounding these are rising healthcare costs, lack of hospital and long-term care beds, and healthcare manpower shortages.

In the face of a healthcare environment that is constantly changing, pharmacy in a comprehensive cancer center needs to be cognizant of new and emerging models of care that are integrated and patient-centered, attentive to cutting-edge research, cancer treatment, and different approaches to managing the entire spectrum of oncological care. To support the functions of a comprehensive cancer center, pharmacy services need to focus on delivering care that is timely and convenient, affordable, financially sustainable, and quality assured.

L. Chew (✉)
Pharmacy, National Cancer Centre Singapore, Singapore, Singapore

Singapore Health Services, Singapore, Singapore

Department of Pharmacy, National University of Singapore, Singapore, Singapore

Chief Pharmacist Office, Ministry of Health, Singapore, Singapore

Singapore Pharmacy Council, Singapore, Singapore
e-mail: lita.chew.s.t@singhealth.com.sg

M. C. M. Thum
Pharmacy, National Cancer Centre Singapore, Singapore, Singapore

Chief Pharmacist Office, Ministry of Health, Singapore, Singapore

© The Author(s) 2022
M. Aljurf et al. (eds.), *The Comprehensive Cancer Center*,
https://doi.org/10.1007/978-3-030-82052-7_9

The prerequisites to transformation from a brick-and-mortar pharmacy model to a progressive pharmacy is guided by the perspectives of (1) investing in people to attract and retain the best, (2) investing in place to build a future-ready facility, (3) investing in process to create greater value for patients, and producing safe and quality products.

The COVID-19 pandemic has brought numerous challenges to the healthcare system. At the same time, it serves as a timely reminder of the importance of pandemic preparedness, not only to support safe and quality use of medicine but ensuring the availability of medicines for patients where and when they need it, as well as the safety and ability of staff to continue to function and respond to disruptions while ensuring the continuity of care for patients.

Investing in People

At the heart of transformation and provision for comprehensive care is a competent healthcare workforce. Pharmacists, as medication experts, are accountable and responsible for promoting safe and effective medication use. As complex cancer care issues continue to demand a multidisciplinary approach, oncology-trained pharmacist is a vital member of the collaborative care team to improve treatment outcomes. The pharmacy department manpower planning needs to move in tandem with prevailing and future cancer care model. It is imperative that the plan takes into consideration a transdisciplinary, shared decision-making practice model as pharmacists expand scope of practice.

Key considerations important to attract and retain a competent pharmacy workforce (pharmacists and pharmacy support staff) include the following:

(a) *A career structure for progression and advancement framework*

Enhancing professional development and competency of existing pharmacy workforce and attracting high potential recruit is a win-win for both employees and employers. In addition to clinical practice track, inclusion of researcher and educator tracks will aid in developing a pool of pharmacists with matrix career tracks such as clinician-researcher and clinician-educator.

(b) *A competency framework to complement the implementation of proposed career pathways*

Taking reference from national, professional and regulatory bodies, the competency framework enables pharmacy workforce to reflect on their practice, identify needs for continuous professional development and acquires new competencies to advance their practice systematically.

A common enabler for workforce transformation in addition to training and development includes but not limited to identifying meaning and purpose, staff engagement, building trust, communication and creating opportunities.

(c) *Manpower and workforce optimization for effective number and skill mix to deliver comprehensive and safe cancer care*

When planning, it is important to consider activity level, service demand and variation, patient acuity, staffing norms, staff experience, organisational service and quality indicators and consistency with published best practices.

Pharmacy technicians form an important part of the pharmacy support workforce. The roles of pharmacy technicians have shifted from picking, packing, dispensing and inventory to support niche areas like medication review, medication administration, information technology support (automation, data analytics), clinical trial drug management and tele-pharmacy. A competency framework from entry to advanced practice would be instrumental to provide a structured approach towards development of this workforce in terms of practice, clinical and task specialization.

(d) *Staff benefits and recognitions*

This can come in the form of training grants and scholarships to fund for further studies and residency training, or competitive staff remuneration package that recognizes high potential and performing individuals.

Investing in Place

Oncology pharmacy services in a comprehensive cancer facility go above and beyond needs to build a future-ready facility. Proper space planning for a pharmacy facility can ensure configurable space when the need arises. COVID-19 pandemic has brought about the creative use of space amidst social distancing requirements. Wherever possible, space reconfigurability, mapping of patient journey, equipment and material flow and processes must be well thought out to ensure workplace continues to support job to be carried out in the most efficient manner.

Key considerations for a future-ready pharmacy in a comprehensive cancer center include the following:

(a) *Adopting technology*

Harnessing new technology such as automation, robotic, and RFID technologies to ensure a highly efficient and accurate medication dispensing process has enabled pharmacy workforce to deliver more valued direct patient care activities. The use of automation and robotics requires careful planning, ensuring workflow marries the capabilities of robotics to seek the best outcome of safety and efficiency for the pharmacy. With the increasing complexity in medication regimes, and array of decision-making tools available, it is crucial to ensure that these tools fit into the overall information technology workflow so that these systems fulfill the purported benefits.

The use of artificial intelligence (AI) can inform patient load and flow, thereby allowing workforce planning and optimization. On the clinical front, use of AI to predict patient response or adverse reactions to a drug is not a far-off reality. Pharmacies must be ready to embrace the wealth of data and turn them into meaningful information to inform practice.

(b) *Good Manufacturing Practice (GMP)*

Sterile compounding is an integral component of a cancer center pharmacy. Quality assurance and control is paramount to ensure that cancer patients receive the right drug in the right dose, at the right time and with right vehicle and container. GMP in the pharmacy laboratory accords patients and providers of sterile compounded products a seal of quality assurance. Fatal incidents have been reported worldwide (e.g. lack of vigilant decision-making process and anticipatory models with programs to prevent errors, disaster and crisis in the New England Compounding Centre leading to fatalities from meningitis from tainted sterile products) [1]. The hub-and-spoke model for sterile compounding in Singapore leveraged on the principles of quality assurance and efficiency to provide the nation with cost-effective and quality sterile products [2]. It is of tactical importance that a comprehensive cancer center pharmacy laboratory becomes a GMP-certified hub.

(c) *Business continuity planning (BCP)*

Identifying risks that has high impact on the business operations is the initial step in formulating the BCP plan. Critical operations and functions that need to be continued are then identified and prioritized [3] . Communicating the plan to key stakeholders is important. A BCP plan once developed and implemented needs to be maintained. Constant drills and refinement should be in place to keep up with the changes in practice.

Investing in Process and New Models of Care

Processes bring people and place together. The aim of achieving optimum process in pharmacy is to deliver seamless integration of pharmacy services into the patient's cancer journey. Pharmacy needs to lead in the medication management process. Organizations with foresight, agility, and resilience recognize the need to continually improve their processes to meet the needs of the changing healthcare landscape and their patients. Research forms the backbone of a comprehensive cancer center. Pharmacy involvement in the new models of care needs to embrace bench to bedside research, including novel therapies (drugs, biologics, and medical devices) and survivorship. The latter is of increasing focus as screening and treatment modalities sees shifting demographics and increased cure options.

Key considerations in process management and improvement include:

(a) *Medication use and procurement*

A good medication management system supports appropriate and judicious use of drugs. Rapid reviews using health technology assessment methodologies are useful tools for presenting evidence-based reviews and expert opinion for decision making. Drug utilization evaluation that assesses the appropriateness of drug use can provide timely feedback and presents evidence for rectification.

To help facilitate the safe, effective, and timely administration of innovative therapies to cancer patients, it will be important for pharmacy to collaborate with clinicians, researchers, educators, and administrators to develop policy and procedure pertaining to approval for access, evidence-based guidance, work instructions, and educational materials for these therapeutics.

Procurement becomes more complicated as cancer care becomes increasingly more individualized and complex with precision medicine and novel treatments, including but not limited to CAR T-cell therapy, novel immunotherapies, and gene targeting approaches.

Similarly, for access to generic drugs and biosimilars, pharmaceutical procurement expertise is needed to ensure timely and relevant input into procurement of generic drugs and biosimilar choices. Fulfilment of contracts, negotiation, and lock-in of preferential drug pricing are other important functions of procurement.

(b) *Medication supply*

From the ordering to administration of medications, numerous processes are involved before medication is supplied. These processes must be engineered and constantly reviewed to ensure effective communication between all parties involved. Strict standards should be set for ordering, preparing, dispensing, administration, handling, and storage of chemotherapy to ensure all important elements are addressed [4].

Presently, home delivery of oral chemotherapy drugs presents an attractive option for patients' convenience, avoids overcrowding in pharmacies, and facilitates round-the-clock access. Patients can wait in the comfort of their homes/offices where the medications will be delivered. Other supply alternatives include express pickup at designated dispensing sites and secure lockers for patients who do not want home delivery option.

(c) *Administration*

There has been increasing focus on delivering care that is centered on the needs and preferences of patients, administered in the most clinically appropriate and convenient settings for patients. Home and community administration of chemotherapy have been made possible with the availability of subcutaneous dosage forms and smart ambulatory infusion devices. A clear set of service guidance and criteria involving multi-stakeholders, including but not limited to clinicians, nursing, clinic operation and business office, need to be established for pharmacy to support the care model.

(d) *Monitoring*

With mobile applications that supports tele-consult, patient-reported outcomes and patient-reported experience, oncology pharmacists can help patients to achieve better medication adherence and monitoring of adverse effects arising from treatment. Research looking at mobile application-based monitoring and intervention, and factors that affect oral chemotherapy adherence, can help to improve medication use process for cancer patients [5].

(e) *Community partnership for cancer education and survivorship*

Pharmacy can support patient and caregiver engagement through development of online patient information leaflets, patient counselling, medication therapy management clinics, tele-pharmacy, and public education seminars.

According to the National Cancer Institute, survivorship starts from the time of diagnosis to the end of life, focusing on the health and well-being of a person with cancer including the physical, mental, emotional, social and financial effects of cancer [6]. Pharmacy can support survivorship initiatives through patient education, pharmacy and nurse-led survivorship programs or clinics, as well as partnering with community pharmacies to support the physical effects of cancer such as nutrition, prosthesis, stoma and dressing supplies.

(f) *Resource optimization*

Pharmacy must work within allocated resources to achieve desired outcomes. Through utilization of visual stream mapping and data analytics to guide day-to-day activities and its variation, for example in chemotherapy scheduling, staff rostering, and medication fulfilment, pharmacy will have the capability to balance and optimize available resources with service demand.

(g) *Quality improvement*

Continuous quality improvement must be embedded into the culture of a future-proof pharmacy. Process improvements can range from small changes in workflow to improve efficiency, to impacting patients' experience in the cancer care journey. Embracing the concept of Kaizen is a good start. It involves applying 'process-oriented thinking', 'plan-do-study-check-act' and 'standardize-do-check-act cycles' approaches, speaking with data, embracing quality-first and focusing on the customer [7]. New processes are also subjected to failure mode effect analysis to identify risk and develop mitigation strategies. Investing in process improvement requires a proactive and concerted effort by staff at all levels. It is important to raise issues promptly and seek timely support for resolution.

Building a Sustainable Pharmacy

From terrorist attacks and cyber threats to hurricane, riots, and pandemic, disrupters abound. Technological disrupters such as the Internet, social media, and AI are also changing the fabric of society. While future events may not take same form, they will require a deliberate effort from organization to navigate with agility and effectively.

Key considerations in building a sustainable pharmacy include:

(a) *Self-sustainability*

The pandemic has highlighted the importance of diverse supply chains. Establishing emergency drug formularies and resolving drug shortages has become a priority in these times. Strong collaborations with the governmental agencies and establishing networks to ensure adequacy of essential medications must complement rational stockpiling and stock rotation to achieve national drug supply objectives. Methods of drug savings through centralized compounding can and should be explored.

Pharmacy ought to support different models of care and work together with other care providers to provide remote pharmacy services through telemedicine and home delivery when the need arises. Empowering patients for self-care and flagging issues to pharmacists and healthcare professionals allows patients to be more involved in their own care, allowing healthcare professionals' limited resources to be used in the most value-added tasks.

Staff well-being, as well as education and training, plays an important role towards self-sustenance. Staff must now cope with disruptions brought about by technological advances as well as new working norms brought about by pandemic. Mental health and staff well-being are thus integral factors to build a sustainable workforce. The pandemic has also changed the delivery of education, and training and new modalities must be explored to ensure staff are upskilled and remain relevant and always ready.

Societal changes and demographic shifts necessitate the adoption of technology, including mobile applications, AI-enabled medication support, robotics, and automation, to sustain pharmacy services and delivery of pharmaceutical care in peace time and during disruption.

(b) *Environmental sustainability*

Interventions for a greener pharmacy include the adoption of a wide array of environmentally friendly activities ranging from facility to practice. Energy-saving ventilation, water, and lighting practices should be encouraged in the facility. The energy consumption of equipment and automation should form part of the evaluation criteria in the procurement process. Proactive scheduling of replacement of older equipment with newer and energy-saving ones should form part of the equipment management process. Pharmacy must strive to encourage recycling, reduce the use of paper through adoption of electronic systems, and decrease reliance on plastics. This will save running costs in the long term and decrease the carbon footprint from these day-to-day activities.

On the practice front, interventions include reducing imprudent prescribing, which can result in stockpiling, improper storage, and irresponsible disposal with the consequences of poisonings, pollution, and wasted healthcare resources [8]. Patient education becomes important to prevent adherence problems arising from lack of understanding of drugs and their side effects and thus wastage of medications. Stockpiling of medications at home should be discouraged through medication reviews and counselling.

Patient education on proper medication disposal, in particular, cancer and targeted therapies, should be part of the patient journey. Pain medications like fentanyl patches can also lead to issues of drug abuse and harm through inadvertent exposure if not disposed properly. Pharmacists are in the prime position to provide advice on the proper handling and disposal of these medications as well as to provide support for proper disposal.

(c) *Financial sustainability*

It is challenging to achieve the right balance across the key priorities of efficiency, safety, quality, accessibility and affordability. To achieve efficiency, safety and quality, pharmacy needs to invest more resources and inject technology in the overall medication management and use. To make accessible innovative and novel therapeutics to patients, pharmacy needs to have sufficient drug budget to procure, while affordability remains questionable depending on who is paying for the costs of treatments. Therefore, an important consideration that underpins these priorities is financial sustainability.

Health technology assessment is an important capability to have, grow and apply in pharmacy, so that new treatments, technologies, and drugs can be evaluated, and judicious decision can be made for availability and access. Given the rapid medical advances, this can help to avoid unnecessary expenditure on new and unproven, or less effective treatment.

Conclusion

Pharmacy in a comprehensive cancer center must be geared to provide comprehensive pharmacy services to a diverse population of cancer patients. The pharmacy workforce consisting of oncology specialty trained pharmacists, generalist pharmacists, pharmacy technicians, administrators, and other support personnel is competent and committed to clinical excellence, continuous process improvement, and innovation in pharmacy practice.

Investment in a modernized pharmacy will lead to improve safety, efficiency, and effectiveness in medication management, distribution, handling of hazardous drugs, and advancement in practice model.

Given the likely increase in demand for cancer care, new therapeutics and the complexity of cancer treatment, it is apparent that high-quality care for cancer patients will require an end-to-end medication use process that is robust and cost-effective, while also helping patients access pharmaceutical care when and where is needed.

Building to last should be the long-term strategic view for a sustainable pharmacy practice model. The need to be nimble and responsive to changes, recognize the need to be innovative and develop new solutions, being eco-conscious and prudence in spending are key ingredients toward better, faster, safer, and enduring pharmacy for the patients we serve.

References

1. Olaniran BA, Scholl JC. New England Compounding Center Meningitis Outbreak: a compounding public health crisis. J Risk Anal Cris Resp. 2014;4(1):34–42.
2. Ministry of Health Singapore. National Pharmacy Strategy. https://www.moh.gov.sg/hpp/pharmacists/national-pharmacy-strategy. Accessed 11 Sept 2020.

3. WHO guidance for business continuity planning. Geneva: World Health Organization; 2018. License: CC BY-NC-SA 3.0 IGO.
4. Neuss MN, Gilmore TR, et al. 2016 Updated American Society of Clinical Oncology/Oncology Nursing Society Chemotherapy Administration Safety Standards, including standards for pediatric oncology. ONF. 2017, 44(1). http://onf.ons.org/onf/44//1/2016-updated-american-society-clinical-oncologyoncology-nursing-society-chemotherapy. Accessed 20 Aug 2020
5. Ali EE, Leow JL, Chew L, Yap KYL. Patients' perception of app-based educational and behavioural interventions for enhancing oral anticancer medication adherence. J Cancer Educ. 2017; https://doi.org/10.1007/s13187-017-1248-x.
6. National Cancer Institute. Survivorship. https://www.cancer.gov/publications/dictionaries/cancer-terms/def/survivorship. Accessed 20 Aug 2020
7. Imai M. Gemba Kaizen. 2nd ed. United States of America: The Kaizen Institute, Ltd, McGraw-Hill; 2012.
8. Daughton CG. Drugs and the environment: stewardship & sustainability. National Exposure Research Laboratory, Environmental Sciences Division, US EPA, Las Vegas, Nevada, report NERL-LVESD 10/081, EPA/600?R-10/106, 12 September 2010, 196 pp, http://www.epa.gov/Exe/ZyPDF.cgi/P1008L3M.PDF?Dockey=P1008L3M.PDF. Accessed 17 Aug 2020.

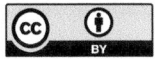

Chapter 10
Administrative Support

Gabriel Alcantara and Nelson J. Chao

Strategic Planning

The capacity to develop a comprehensive cancer center varies with available resources such as human capital (providers, nurses, staff), facilities and equipment, and most importantly financial funding. The availability of such resources will dictate the services that can be provided. Sources of funding vary widely and can include national and subnational government funding; private user payments, either through health insurance or out of pocket, revenue-generating practices such as retail and parking, and philanthropic support from external donors. Strategic planning allows for a proactive approach in determining what populations can be served, what services can be delivered, the funding needs to grow the center, and developing and directing a short- and long-term business plan for expansion, implementation, and sustainability.

The long-term financial health of a cancer center ultimately determines its ability to effectively deliver quality cancer care services. Thus, another key component in strategic planning is the ability to understand the market intelligence and the ability to change as market conditions change. Changes in market conditions include changes in governmental funding; changes in private payer policies and practices; pricing changes for medical supplies, equipment, and personnel; and even scientific development and the subsequent delivery of new cancer treatments. The impact of such changes needs to then be evaluated within the context of the socio-demographics and health needs of the patient population that the cancer center is looking to serve.

G. Alcantara (✉)
Duke Cancer Institute, Duke University Department of Medicine, Division of Hematologic Malignancies & Cellular Therapy, Durham, NC, USA
e-mail: gabriel.alcantara@duke.edu

N. J. Chao
Division of Hematologic Malignancies and Cellular Therapy/BMT, Global Cancer/Duke Cancer Institute/Duke Global Health Institute, Durham, NC, USA

M. Aljurf et al. (eds.), *The Comprehensive Cancer Center*,
https://doi.org/10.1007/978-3-030-82052-7_10

Effective planning and understanding of the culminating effect of these various factors will enable a cancer center to grow strategically in a manner that is fiscally responsible and positions it well for sustainability.

Space and Facilities Planning and Program Development

Strategic planning eventually transforms into program development and the operational execution of such plans to enable safe, quality, and efficient patient care. Administrative personnel are often responsible for the design of physical spaces as well as design of workflows and processes to move patients through the various steps in their care. If the strategic planning team can identify the volume of the patient population that needs to be served, then the administrative team can plan the type and number of resources needed to provide comprehensive cancer care:

- Number of inpatient beds
- Number of outpatient exam rooms
- Number of surgical suites
- Number of infusion chairs for outpatient treatment
- Number of radiation therapy machines
- Number of imaging machines
- Number of lab draw stations
- Number of waiting room chairs
- Number of parking spaces
- Time it takes for lab results
- Time it takes for chemotherapy to be prepared
- Time it takes for an inpatient bed to be turned
- Time it takes for an outpatient exam room to be turned
- Time it takes for a patient to enter/exit the cancer center (cycle time)

Coupled with human resource planning, such space planning is necessary to ensure that your cancer center facility is designed and built to efficiently manage the patient demand.

Financial Management

All cancer centers need administrative support and competent financial systems to monitor and manage revenues and expenses of the centers. Centers need competent financial and accounting systems that measure the collective productivity of the center – the units of service being administered, the number of patient visits, etc., and the relationship of expenses to incoming revenue for the delivery of such services.

Healthy revenue management and enhancement is maintained by instituting and improving policies and processes to assure all clinical services are billed accurately and timely, and that collections are pursued promptly and accurately. Retrospective analysis of charge capture, denial reasons, and reimbursement patterns can result in recommended actions to optimize the revenue return. Such action could include developing guidelines, providing feedback, and educating providers and staff on billing processes and practices that accurately reflect the level of service being delivered and that maximize the financial return for such service or even the movement or services to a lower cost setting or delivery of new services that may have more long-term reduction in health-care expense – all of which is also a factor of strategic planning.

Budgeting

Administrative support is also needed for the management of expenses – budgeting of personnel and non-personnel expenses for operating purposes and how they relate to anticipated patient volumes and revenue expectations. Capital budgets are needed for the planning of financial reserves for the larger capital purchases such as equipment, furniture, and maintenance, acquisition, or construction of facilities.

There may be instances where the patient revenue stream from private payers, governmental payers, or self-pay patients does not cover all the expenses necessary to deliver the needed health-care services. If such is the case, then alternative sources of revenue should be sought such as grants or philanthropic support from financial donors or even a form of subsidization from the larger institution or health system. In all cases, obtaining of such financial support typically requires the development of a business plan that explains to the investor(s) the mission of the cancer center, the long-term goal it aims to accomplish, and the level of investment and support needed to carry out such mission. Effective management of sponsored funds and philanthropic support require an additional level of accountability in complying and adhering the spending as per the conditions of the sponsor or donor.

Performance Management

A growing concern today is the overall cost of health care. There are changes occurring today to improve the "value" of health care begging to ask the question of "am I getting the best quality care at the best price?" A comprehensive cancer center needs an administrative infrastructure to measure the overall performance of the center – in quality and outcomes, patient volumes, patient satisfaction, workforce satisfaction, and financial performance. It is important to be able to measure quality outcomes in both acute and long-term setting. Acute quality measures for cancer hospitals typically include infection rates, length of stay, readmission rates, and mortality rates. Acute quality measures in the ambulatory setting are a bit more limited and are typically measured more by operational measures such as patient satisfaction (were the needs of the patient met?) and cycle time (measure of throughput for time the patient spends at cancer center and its various services). Overall, the healthcare industry is moving towards improved measures that measure overall health over the patient's care continuum vs measuring episodic moments such as outpatient visits and hospital stays on an individual basis. This level of value-based care will require enhanced collaborations across various specialties beyond hematology/oncology to address the adverse health impacts that may come with the delivery of cancer treatments (cardio or neuro toxicities, for instance) as well as primary care in the survivorship setting, and marriage and family therapy to address the psychosocial and mental health impacts that come with cancer care. In this ever-changing market, administrative support is needed to be able to report on such performance outcomes so that centers can gauge their effectiveness and efficiency in the delivery of care and make internal adjustments as needed.

Regulatory and Accreditation Standards

Yet another component of performance management is the evaluation of the healthcare provider's ability to provide safe and effective care of the highest quality and value per the standards of regulatory and accreditation agencies. Specially trained administrative support with regulatory knowledge is needed in a comprehensive cancer center to ensure compliance to regulatory and accreditation standards that are required for the provision of clinical services. Such accreditations can range from overall delivery, quality, and environment of health care – in the USA for instance, the Joint Commission on Accreditation of Healthcare Organizations (JCAHO) is responsible for the accreditation of all healthcare organizations. However, cancer services may also require more specialized accreditations for services such as chemotherapy, radiation therapy, clinical laboratories, and transplantation and cellular therapy.

Human Resources Management

- Refining and developing the administrative structure that provides the necessary level of support services for the sustainable growth and success of the center
- Understanding and appropriately implementing the varied policies and procedures for providers and staff
- Generally overseeing personnel actions for providers and staff such as recruitment, selecting and hiring, training, performance management, promotions, succession planning, and terminations

Access Services

A core administrative service of any comprehensive cancer center is the access function – the intake or management of new patients into the cancer center via self-referrals or physician referrals. Referrals can come in from a variety of sources – telephone, fax, or internal via the electronic medical record system. Key administrative components of an access team include:

- Utilization of scheduling questionnaires/algorithms to appropriately triage patient
- Insurance verification
- Medical record collection
- Referral management (inbound and outbound)

Scheduling Questionnaires

Scheduling questionnaires ought to be developed to guide the scheduler through a series of questions designed to assign the patient to the right provider at the right time for an appropriate diagnosis. For example:

1. What is the reason for your call or visit? Is this a new diagnosis, existing diagnosis, a relapse or refractory diagnosis, a second opinion, or establishment of long-term follow-up care?
2. For solid tumors, do you need to see a medical oncologist, surgical oncologist, radiation oncologist, or all three?
3. For blood cancers, do you need to see a hematologist/oncologist or do you need to see a stem cell transplant specialist?

The patient or referring physician's office personnel may not always fully understand what services they are in need of given their unfamiliarity with the disease. In such cases, scheduling questionnaires can help guide schedulers through the appropriate questions to determine what services may be needed next. For example, does the patient have a definitive diagnosis from a pathology record? If not, has the patient been scheduled for a surgical biopsy to obtain a specimen for pathology to analyze and diagnose? Based on the information gathered, the scheduler utilizes the scheduling questionnaire and a diagnosis algorithm to assign them to an appropriate oncologist for that condition. Given the rapid and escalating potential of a cancer diagnosis, every effort should be made to have a patient seen timely; a goal of many comprehensive cancer centers is to offer patients an appointment in as soon as 72 hours or 7 days or less is another common goal. Some more chronic conditions can wait to be seen a bit further out, that is, a few weeks out. The challenge there is managing the anxiety that often comes with a patient waiting to understand their new condition and eager to learn what is next. Some cancer access teams utilize a nurse or patient navigator to help review the patient's medical records to ensure if they can in fact wait to be seen, but a nurse in such role can help a patient waiting to be seen understand their condition and help them navigate what is often a complicated network of various specialties to diagnose, treat, and manage a cancer diagnosis.

Insurance Verification and Medical Record Collection

Depending on the financial clearance policies of your cancer center, protocols may need to be established to ensure that new patients have a financial plan to pay for their cancer services, whether that be through self-pay or through insurance. Uninsured or underinsured patients may need another mitigation strategy such as referral to another center that accepts their insurance, financial assistance from the center, or assistance in applying for governmental or foundational support for their care. Though not common, there could also be the scenario of a patient needing immediate emergency or urgent care – in such cases, the goal is to provide the appropriate clinical services to stabilize the patient while other financial options continue to be explored.

Assuming the patient meets the financial and medical clearance to be seen by the oncology team, various medical records are collected from the referring provider office and other medical offices that may have participated in the patient's care over the years. The goal of such record collection is to ensure that the oncologist has as much comprehensive clinical information. Medical records that may or may not need to be collected in advance of the patient visit include:

- Physician notes
- History and physical
- Diagnosing or relapse pathology
- Cytogenetic reports
- Flow cytometry
- Lab results
- Imaging results (CT/MRI/PET/US)
- Screening results (mammography, colonoscopy, PAP smear)
- Chemotherapy flow sheets (hospital and clinic)
- Radiation treatment summaries
- Operative reports
- Medication list

Referral Management

Comprehensive cancer centers are becoming increasingly aware that access services are maturing from just scheduling to more enhanced referral management. Referral management is defined as the process by which patients are transitioned to the next step in their care. Normally, referral management takes place when a condition changes for the patient, thus necessitating a referral to a specialist but there are various cases in which care may also be appropriate to transition out or be shared, for example:

- Patients who are in remission and can be transitioned to a survivorship program or care with their primary care physician
- Patients who can receive part of most of their oncologic care closer to home

- Patients with complex conditions who may require various specialties in addition to hematology/oncology, that is, cardiology, neurology, rheumatology, endocrinology

The plan for when to make those transitions of care is planned by the oncologist, but a strong, clerical administrative group is essential in making these transitions back and forth across various care settings – it can often be a high-volume, busy function requiring the ability to multi-task and be organized in managing the various patients being referring in and out. This necessitates a key customer service ingredient – relationship management – the cancer center's access and scheduling teams are often the first and the lifeline connecting the various medical offices, and thus it is critical to ensure smooth and efficient processes so as not to delay care. As more options present for cancer care, a strong referral base may choose to refer their patients elsewhere when cancer centers have processes and policies that make it difficult for patients to access.

Conclusion

In summary, a solid administrative infrastructure is necessary for a comprehensive cancer center to efficiently and effectively deliver cancer care. From intake/access functions to high-level strategic planning for the future, such administrative functions are needed to keep the cancer center solvent and well positioned to meet the needs of our cancer patients.

References

1. Fawthrop M. An administrator's guide to departments of internal medicine. 5th ed; 2017.
2. Gelband H, Jha P, Sankaranarayanan R, et al. Cancer: disease control priorities, vol. 3. 3rd ed. Washington, DC; 2015. https://www.ncbi.nlm.nih.gov/books/NBK343637/
3. Gospodarowicz M, Trypuc J, et al. Chapter 11: Cancer Services and the Comprehensive Cancer Center.
4. Healthcare Management Degree Guide. What is JCAHO?. 2020. https://www.healthcare-management-degree.net/faq/what-is-jcaho/.
5. Woodstock E. Patient access symposium 2017 report – Compilation of interviews. 2017.

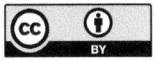

Chapter 11
Psychosocial and Patient Support Services in Comprehensive Cancer Centers

Rajshekhar Chakraborty, Navneet S. Majhail, and Jame Abraham

Introduction

As the number of cancer survivors continues to increase due to a rising cancer incidence, better treatment, and early detection, there is a growing need for comprehensive psychosocial and supportive care at comprehensive cancer centers. Based on cancer incidence and survival statistics in the United States, the number of cancer survivors will increase to 20 million by 2026 [1]. Supportive care services not only benefit patients who are cured or have achieved long-term remission, but also those living with metastatic disease. However, despite current guidelines on survivorship care, many recommendations have not been uniformly implemented across cancer centers. For example, in a survey conducted by the American Psychological Oncology Society [APOS], approximately half of the clinical cancer centers did not offer routine psychosocial screening for new cancer patients [2]. The Institute of Medicine [IOM] has also framed several key recommendations to ensure that cancer survivors are not lost in transition after completing active treatment [3]. Hence, strategically addressing both psychosocial and physical effects in cancer survivors should be an important treatment goal that needs to be uniformly addressed by comprehensive cancer centers [4]. In this chapter, we will discuss the key psychosocial

R. Chakraborty (✉)
Columbia University Medical Center, New York, NY, USA
e-mail: rc3360@cumc.columbia.edu

N. S. Majhail
Blood and Marrow Transplant Program, Department of Hematology-Oncology, Cleveland Clinic Taussig Cancer Center, Cleveland, OH, USA
e-mail: navneet.majhail@sarahcannon.com

J. Abraham
Department of Hematology-Oncology, Cleveland Clinic Taussig Cancer Center, Cleveland, OH, USA
e-mail: abrahaj5@ccf.org

© The Author(s) 2022
M. Aljurf et al. (eds.), *The Comprehensive Cancer Center*,
https://doi.org/10.1007/978-3-030-82052-7_11

and supportive care services that are required as a part of survivorship programs at comprehensive cancer centers. We will discuss the services required for managing common psychosocial and physical effects experienced by cancer survivors and the current models of survivorship care. Pharmacologic management of psychosocial and physical issues in cancer survivors are outside the scope of this chapter and will not be discussed here. Palliative care and hospice are an important component of comprehensive cancer care and are discussed in detail in Chap. 9. Table 11.1 describes various domains that fall within the purview of cancer center patient support services and psychosocial care and the resources recommended for their effective management.

Common Psychosocial and Physical Effects

Distress and Mood Disorders

The National Comprehensive Cancer Network (NCCN) defines distress as an unpleasant experience of psychological, social, spiritual, and/or physical nature that may hinder the ability of patients to cope effectively with cancer or its treatment [5]. Distress is prevalent in approximately one-third of cancer survivors and can be associated with a reduced quality of life [6, 7]. Furthermore, patients experiencing distress have a lower likelihood of adhering to recommended health behaviors and surveillance strategies [8]. Mood disorders, including anxiety, depression, or post-traumatic stress disorder [PTSD] is also prevalent among cancer survivors and warrants screening by the oncologist or primary care physician [PCP] [4]. A meta-analysis showed the odds ratio of PTSD in cancer survivors to be 1.66 compared to controls [9].

Screening for distress, anxiety, and depression is recommended by the NCCN survivorship guidelines. The NCCN distress thermometer along with other tools such as PHQ9 can be easily administered prior to clinic visit such that the clinician and appropriate support staff [e.g., social worker or financial navigator] can be notified.

Services Required for Management

Patients who display signs of anxiety, depression, or distress on initial screening should be thoroughly evaluated by the oncologist regarding any physical cause related to cancer or anticancer therapy. Furthermore, safety evaluation, such as suicidal intent, safety at home, and social isolation, should be conducted by appropriate personnel. Access to licensed social workers experienced in caring for cancer patients or a dedicated psycho-oncologist is desirable for initial evaluation prior to referring

Table 11.1 Various domains of services for patient support and psychosocial care within comprehensive cancer centers

Domain	Personnel support	Infrastructure support
Advance care planning	Social worker	Clinic space
Care coordination	Care coordinators, patient navigators, nurse navigators	Clinic space, technology support to facilitate care coordination
Community outreach	Care coordinators, social worker, patient navigator	Cancer screening, infrastructure to facilitate referral and access to care, outreach programs for underserved populations, community education
Complementary medicine	Providers for specific services (e.g., art and music therapist, yoga instructor)	Space and equipment for services (e.g., yoga, art therapy, music therapy, acupuncture)
Fertility	Gynecologist, urologist, reproductive endocrinologist	Mechanism for counseling and referral for fertility preservation
Financial support and navigation	Financial coordinator, care coordinator, social worker	Workspace, access to extramural and community services and grants, assistance for local housing
Genetic counseling	Genetic counselors	Clinic space
Home care services	Patient navigator, social worker, nurse	Infrastructure to provide lab services, medication administration, and other care at home
Pain and symptom management	Palliative care physician/advance practice provider and nurse, physical therapist, occupational therapist, rehabilitation medicine provider, nutrition therapist	Clinic space, space and equipment for rehabilitation services, liaison with hospice services
Patient information and education	Patient navigator, nurse coordinator, social worker	Patient resource library, information technology support for patient education, workspace, and meeting rooms
Pharmacy	Pharmacist	Pharmacy space, supply chain to provide access to chemotherapeutic and supportive care drugs.
Psychological assessment and support	Social worker, psychiatrist, psychologist, spiritual care providers (e.g., chaplain)	Clinic space, technology support for assessments, support groups, access to community resources for psychological support, liaison with other psychiatric services in the institution
Special populations (e.g., pediatric, adolescent, young adult, and geriatric patients)	Clinical providers with expertise in treating specific patient populations	Clinic space, other support services geared specifically towards special populations

(continued)

Table 11.1 (continued)

Domain	Personnel support	Infrastructure support
Special services (e.g., post-laryngectomy, ostomy care, speech pathology)	Physician, advance practice provider, nurse, or other providers based on need	Clinic space, equipment, and other support based on specific scenario
Survivorship care	Advance practice providers or nurses, social worker, specialists, patient navigator, care coordinator	Clinic space, resources for patient education, resources for generating and provision of survivorship care plan

selected patients to psychiatry. Access to a psychiatrist who specializes in the care of cancer survivors is desirable. There is robust evidence for several non-pharmacological measures for the treatment of distress and mood disorders. Several meta-analyses have demonstrated beneficial effect of exercise on overall reduction in depressive symptoms among cancer survivors [10, 11]. Hence, providing services and transportation for a structured exercise program to selected patients can be beneficial and improve their quality of life. Cognitive-behavioral therapy [CBT] is effective for the treatment of PTSD in general population [12], and is also recommended for cancer survivors with PTSD [4]. Data on the efficacy of integrative medicine in improving the mental health of cancer survivors is limited. However, mindfulness-based stress reduction [MBSR] has the highest quality evidence on improving mental health in breast cancer survivors. A randomized controlled trial [RCT] on 322 breast cancer survivors showed that patients undergoing MBSR had improvement in psychological symptoms of anxiety, fear of recurrence, and fatigue compared to usual care, with the magnitude of benefit being greatest among patients with highest levels of baseline stress [13]. Notably, the intervention consisted of weekly 2-hour sessions for 6 weeks conducted by a clinical psychologist trained in MBSR, with the meditative practices consisting of sitting meditation, walking meditation, body scan, and gentle *Hatha Yoga*. Similar results have been replicated by other RCTs as well [14–16]. Hence, providing integrative and lifestyle medicine services to cancer survivors can be beneficial, especially for those with distress due to fear of recurrence or persistent fatigue. Online or distance sessions should also be provided for patients who cannot attend in person due to logistical reasons. At the Cleveland Clinic's Taussig Cancer Center, we provide free *Yoga* classes by a certified yoga instructor and a registered nurse. Furthermore, the Integrative and Lifestyle Medicine Institute at the Cleveland Clinic also provides classes on *Yoga* and mindfulness meditation.

Fatigue

Fatigue in cancer survivors is defined as emotional, physical, or cognitive tiredness as a result of cancer or its treatment that can interfere with activities of daily living [4]. The putative mechanisms for cancer-related fatigue are pro-inflammatory state, dysregulation of hypothalamic-pituitary-adrenal axis, skeletal muscle wasting, genetics, and psychosocial/ behavioral factors, among others [17]. A large study on cancer survivors from the PROFILES registry showed a high incidence of fatigue at 39–51% among cancer survivors, depending on the tumor type [18]. Persistent fatigue can lead to impaired health-related quality of life [HRQoL] and a decreased likelihood of staying employed [4]. The NCCN guidelines recommend that oncologists should screen cancer survivors for fatigue, based on patients' description of their fatigue level. Several patient-reported questionnaires such as Brief Fatigue Inventory [BFI] are also available that can be used for screening [19].

Services Required for Management

The first step in the management of fatigue is to identify and treat the contributing factors, if any, such as pain, nausea, or dyspnea [4]. An RCT from the Netherlands showed superiority of nurse-led monitoring and treatment of physical symptoms over usual care in alleviating fatigue as well as interference of fatigue with daily living in cancer survivors [20]. The symptoms that were of major concern to fatigued patients were pain, shortness of breath, and decreased appetite.

Increasing physical activity has category 1 recommendation for the management of fatigue in cancer survivors [4]. A Cochrane systematic review had studied the impact of exercise on cancer-related fatigue, as observed in RCTs [21]. At the end of study intervention period, patients who were randomized to exercise intervention had significantly lower fatigue compared to those in the control arm, especially in breast and prostate cancer survivors [21]. Subsequently, another large meta-analysis compared exercise, psychological, and pharmaceutical treatments for the treatment of cancer-related fatigue [22]. Interestingly, exercise, exercise plus psychological, and psychological interventions all led to a statistically significant as well as clinically meaningful decrease in fatigue at the end of intervention period, whereas pharmaceutical interventions did not. The absolute mean weighted effect size was numerically highest with exercise intervention [22]. Referral to a physical therapist or an exercise specialist should be strongly considered for cancer survivors who are at a risk of injury, for example, survivors with bone metastasis.

Several psychosocial and behavioral interventions, such as MBSR, CBT, psychoeducational therapy, support groups, and journal writing, have shown promise in the treatment of cancer-related fatigue. A meta-analysis of RCTs on behavioral and psychosocial interventions showed a statistically significant reduction in fatigue, depression, anxiety, and stress [23]. Acupuncture is also considered to be an acceptable option for cancer-related fatigue; however, data from RCTs have been conflicting thus far [24, 25].

Pain

Pain is one of the most concerning symptoms that is prevalent in approximately one-third of cancer survivors and can lead to depression, lack of sleep, and poor quality of life [26]. There is a diverse etiology of pain in cancer survivors, including arthralgia in breast cancer patients on aromatase inhibitors and neuropathic pain in patients with chemotherapy-induced peripheral neuropathy. The NCCN guidelines recommend periodic screening for pain in all survivors. Survivors with chronic pain should have easy access to pain management or palliative care specialists under a shared care model. The non-pharmacologic management strategies with a robust evidence base and the services required are summarized below.

Services Required for Management

Several behavioral approaches have been studied for pain management in a randomized fashion. In breast cancer survivors with late post-treatment pain, an 8-week mindfulness-based cognitive intervention led to a significantly decreased pain intensity, nonprescription pain medication use, and improved quality of life compared to usual care in an RCT [27]. Another RCT of sedative music therapy from Taiwan showed a significant decrease in post-intervention pain [28]. Other psychosocial support and behavioral interventions that have been shown to be effective in alleviating cancer-related pain are breathing exercises, relaxation, guided imagery, and hypnosis [29, 30]. There is a high-level evidence for increased physical activity and exercise in the management of cancer-related pain. An RCT of exercise intervention [including aerobic exercise and supervised strength training] in breast cancer survivors with aromatase inhibitor-induced arthralgia showed a significantly lower worst pain score, pain severity, and interference with activities of daily living at the end of 12-month period in the exercise arm [31]. A *Yoga* intervention for cancer survivors also showed decrease in musculoskeletal symptoms, including general pain, muscle ache, and physical discomfort among breast cancer survivors in an RCT [32].

Given pain being highly prevalent in cancer survivors, comprehensive cancer centers should consider provision of these services, including access to physical therapist or an exercise specialist, and classes for several behavioral interventions like mindfulness or relaxation techniques.

Cognitive Dysfunction

Cognitive dysfunction is a well-described long-term side effect of cytotoxic chemotherapy and is associated with impaired functioning and quality of life [33]. An online survey named LIVESTRONG 2010 was conducted between June 2010 and March 2011 on 3108 post-treatment cancer survivors to investigate perceived cognitive dysfunction and depressive symptoms [34]. Approximately one-half of respondents reported current perceived cognitive dysfunction, with the highest prevalence among brain tumor survivors. Notably, perceived cognitive dysfunction was associated with receiving chemotherapy and self-reported depressive symptoms. The current NCCN guidelines acknowledge the lack of effective screening tool for cognitive dysfunction and recommends clinicians to use their judgement and perform appropriate workup in patients who self-report cognitive dysfunction. Several questions that can assess patients' ability to perform activities of daily living and instrumental activities of daily living may help clinicians uncover subtle cognitive dysfunction.

Services Required for Management

Apart from simple non-pharmacological interventions such as deprescribing unnecessary medications and instruction in self-management, robust data on efficacy of behavioral interventions are lacking. In a small RCT, cognitive behavioral therapy [CBT] was shown to improve spiritual well-being and verbal memory in breast cancer survivors but did not have any impact on self-reported daily cognitive complaints [35]. Another small RCT of videoconference-delivered CBT in breast cancer survivors showed significant improvement in perceived cognitive function and neuropsychological processing speed compared to controls who received supportive care [36]. Similar to its impact on other psychosocial and physical effects, structured exercise program offers benefit to patients with cognitive dysfunction as well, with a dose-response relationship observed with greater levels of physical activity [37]. Other services that can offer benefit to patients with cognitive dysfunction include cognitive training [38], relaxation, meditation [39], and *Yoga* [40].

Services for Healthy Lifestyle in Cancer Survivors

Maintaining a healthy lifestyle in cancer survivors, including regular physical activity, a balanced diet, and avoiding tobacco smoking, is associated with superior outcomes in several tumor types [41–43]. There is a robust evidence on the impact of physical activity in reducing the risk of cardiovascular events in cancer survivors. Data from the Childhood Cancer Survivors Study demonstrated the impact of exercise on cardiovascular events in Hodgkin Lymphoma survivors at a median follow-up of approximately 12 years [44]. Furthermore, the impact of exercise was dose-dependent, with the risk of cardiovascular events being significantly lower among patients reporting ≥9 METs [metabolic equivalent hours]/week. Similar results were seen among patients with nonmetastatic breast cancer [45]. The current NCCN guidelines recommend periodic assessment of physical activity level in cancer survivors. A questionnaire survey of 975 cancer survivors identified several barriers for physical activity, including lack of time, lack of access to an exercise environment, uncertainty regarding safety of exercise post-cancer treatment, physical limitations, and lack of knowledge regarding appropriate physical activities [46]. Hence, providing access to a formal exercise program within comprehensive cancer centers can be beneficial to patients and help provide an individualized exercise plan to survivors. Offering behavioral strategies, including telephone counselling, print material on benefits of physical activity, and motivational interviews can also be helpful in increasing physical activity among cancer survivors. Providing tailored print materials to cancer survivors by mail, promoting consumption of fruits and vegetables, reducing fat intake, and increasing exercise has been shown to be superior to providing standardized non-tailored materials in an RCT [47]. At Taussig Cancer Center, we also provide a mentoring program for cancer survivors called as *4th Angel Patient and Caregiver Mentoring Program*, as a part of which, patients and their caregivers are connected with similar cancer survivors who can share their experiences and provide emotional and spiritual guidance.

Survivorship Care Models

A "model" for providing survivorship care is defined as a comprehensive approach for follow-up care of survivors, which can be performed by the oncology team or primary care providers or both [48]. Designing a strategy for caring for long-term cancer survivors is an integral part of most comprehensive cancer centers and has been endorsed by the American Society of Clinical Oncology [48]. A large systematic review has demonstrated that cancer survivors benefit from coordinated posttreatment psychosocial, rehabilitative, and supportive care [48]. Table 11.2 provides guidance on various elements and domains of cancer survivorship care that cancer centers should strive to achieve.

Table 11.2 Various aspects of survivorship care provided by comprehensive cancer centers

Survivorship care elements
Surveillance for cancer recurrence
Monitoring for and management of medical late effects
Monitoring quality of life and management of psychological effects
Screening for secondary malignancies
Providing health education about diagnosis, exposures, and risks for potential late effects
Familial genetic cancer risk assessment
Education about diet, exercise, and healthy living
Management of financial toxicity
Care coordination with primary care physicians/advance practice providers and specialists
Models of survivorship care[a]
Oncology specialist care (follow-up care in oncology setting with treating oncologist)
Multidisciplinary survivorship clinic (care provided by a specialized team in a separate clinical area)
Disease or treatment-specific survivorship clinic (e.g., clinic specifically for blood and marrow transplant survivors)
General survivorship clinic (care provided by physician or advance practice provider that may be in a cancer center or community practice setting)
Consultative survivorship clinic (one-time visit to a physician or advance practice provider to address survivorship issues)
Integrated survivorship clinic (clinic embedded within a treatment focused oncology setting)
Community generalist model (survivorship care provided by primary care physician or advanced practice provider)

[a]According to American Society of Clinical Oncology (https://www.asco.org/practice-policy/cancer-care-initiatives/prevention-survivorship/survivorship/survivorship-3; accessed 09/01/2020)

Survivorship care models are usually described by the type of survivors [tumor-specific versus general], care setting [separate survivorship clinic versus integrated model], type of clinician(s) providing survivorship care [physician-led versus nurse-led versus nurse practitioner-led versus shared-care model], or the purpose of the survivorship program [e.g., transition clinic model] [48]. The Institute of Medicine recommendations have identified four key domains of survivorship care: prevention, surveillance, intervention, and coordination [3]. To our knowledge, there are three large randomized controlled trials that empirically tested different survivorship care models. Wattchow et al from Australia randomized patients with early stage colon cancer who had underwent curative-intent surgery followed by postsurgical chemotherapy to follow-up by general practitioners [primary care] or surgeons [secondary care] for five years, with the prescribed frequency being every three months for the first two years followed by every two months for the subsequent three years [49]. The primary outcome measures, which were measured at 12 and 24 months, were (a) physical and mental quality of life (b) anxiety and depression, and (c) patient satisfaction. At both 12 and 24 months, there was not any clinically meaningful or statistically significant difference in the primary endpoints between the two care groups. Furthermore, the recurrence rate, time to recurrence detection, and death rate were also similar in both groups. Another Canadian study randomized early stage breast cancer survivors who had completed adjuvant chemotherapy +/− radiotherapy to follow-up by the cancer center [CC group] or their own family physician [FP group]. Of note, patients were allowed to receive hormonal therapy during the study period [50]. The primary outcome of the study was rate of recurrence-related serious clinical events, and the secondary outcome was health-related quality of life. There was no difference in the primary or secondary outcomes in either group. The total number of breast cancer recurrences and deaths was similar in both groups. Notably, family physicians in this study were provided follow-up guidelines, including frequency of follow-up, yearly mammogram, diagnostic tests to investigate signs or symptoms of new primary cancers, and close surveillance for vaginal bleeding in patients on tamoxifen. Hence, based on these two studies, a transition clinic model of survivorship care, which focuses on transition of care from specialists to PCPs, should provide results comparable to continued survivorship care at cancer centers, as long as PCPs are provided specific guidance and expectations regarding long-term toxicities, late effects, and signs of disease recurrence. In a survey of PCPs caring for adult survivors of hematopoietic cell transplantation [HCT] in the United States, commonly identified barriers to care delivery were lack of resources to facilitate care, lack of awareness regarding screening/prevention guidelines in HCT survivors, lack of awareness regarding psychosocial needs, inadequate time, and preference of patients to follow-up with their oncologists [51]. Several of these factors can be potentially addressed by providing education, tools for clinical decision making, and guidelines to PCPs caring for cancer survivors. Finally, a third RCT assessed the cost of follow-up in breast cancer survivors by randomizing them into four different treatment schedules [52]. The four schedules differed either in the frequency of visits [every third or sixth month] or in the intensity of diagnostic tests [on a routine basis versus specific clinical grounds]. Neither increasing the visit frequency to every three months nor performing routine diagnostic examinations led to any benefit in disease-free or overall survival despite increasing the cost of care.

Providing patients and their PCPs with a survivorship care plan [SCP] has been endorsed as a key component of survivor care by the Institute of Medicine [3]. However, the evidence on impact of SCPs on health outcomes and health care delivery is conflicting. A large systematic review including 13 randomized studies on SCPs showed largely negative results regarding impact on physical, psychological, and functional well-being, which were the most commonly assessed outcomes [53]. On the other hand, positive findings on proximal outcomes such as the amount of information received, care satisfaction, and physician implementation of recommended care was noted in some studies. One of the major limitations of this review was heterogeneity in study design. A study conducted at ten cancer centers within the NCI-funded Cancer Research Network in the United States showed that oncology and primary care were jointly responsible for the care of cancer survivors, similar to a shared-care model [54]. However, only two out of ten sites had a formal survivorship program in place. Issues with patient finances and insurance reimbursement were also a major area of concern. At the Cleveland Clinic Blood and Marrow Transplant department, we have established a formal survivorship program since 2016 [55]. Since BMT survivors have unique health care needs due to late effects like chronic graft versus host disease, infections, and second cancers, lifelong follow-up and monitoring is recommended according to most guidelines, which prompted us to develop the survivorship program. A shared-care model, in which BMT physician and PCP liaise to provide ongoing care along with referral to other subspecialty services when needed, was thought to be the most appropriate for this patient population. The program consists of day 100 and 1-year survivorship visit by NP, a treatment summary, and care plan developed by the NP on day 100 and 1-year post-transplant for all non-relapsed patients, and development of educational materials. At the 1-year visit, the NP provides patients, their PCPs, and the primary BMT physician with a summary of test results and a revised care plan, which includes recommended screening/preventative guidelines. Hence, development of a successful survivorship program requires several elements, including appropriate consideration of patient and disease-related factors, buy-in from department leadership, allocation of sufficient resources and personnel, and finally, identifying physician champions in different specialties which will be involved in patient care. Finally, as seen in a recent review [48], survivorship care models are highly institution-dependent, which highlights the need for further research in this area to identify optimal care models.

Community Outreach

Finally, comprehensive cancer centers should also engage in community outreach to especially target high-risk population with the goal of early cancer detection to improve outcome. Cleveland Clinic Cancer Center offers cancer prevention, screening, education and navigation programs designed to meet the needs of the diverse community we serve.

We work with local churches, schools, and other nongovernmental organizations. Our partnership with Federally Qualified Health Centers (FQHC) to provide screening services is very unique. Since there are data on delay in cancer treatment initiation among minorities and low-income population [56], our goal is to reduce the disparity by providing preventative education, cancer risk assessments, and recommended screening including mammogram, prostate exam, colonoscopy, low-dose chest CT, and oral cancer screening for appropriate population. If cancer is found, our Cleveland Clinic Cancer Center community outreach patient navigators can also help with providing cancer education and resources, scheduling appointments, arranging transportation, navigating treatments, providing support during appointments, and offering financial guidance.

Patient Support and Psychosocial Services in Resource-Limited Settings

Provision of patient support and psychosocial services (see Table 11.1) are an essential component of comprehensive cancer care. Although not directly related to treatment of underlying cancer, they ultimately impact patient access to care and optimal outcomes. Cancer centers in resource-limited setting should strive to provide these services to patients while recognizing and prioritizing services that are most relevant to their local patients and communities. For example, in areas where cancer care is largely subsidized by the government, there may not be much need for personnel who need to focus on financial navigation for patients. On the other hand, some elements comprise basic cancer care and should be considered in the planning phase of developing a cancer center such that personnel and infrastructure investments can be made early on. Examples of such services include social work, palliative care, and survivorship care. In several resource-limited settings, local and regional health care in areas other cancer may be better developed – an attempt should be made to identify, optimize, and share existing resources. In these settings, cancer care is often provided by the government and advocating with policy makers to emphasize the importance of psychosocial and patient support services often needed to ensure sufficient resources and infrastructure is assigned towards their development. Ultimately a needs assessment is required as a cancer center is being established with the plan to bring in these services early and focus on domains that will have the most impact on patients and local communities.

References

1. Miller KD, Siegel RL, Lin CC, et al. Cancer treatment and survivorship statistics, 2016. CA Cancer J Clin. 2016;66(4):271–89.
2. Deshields T, Zebrack B, Kennedy V. The state of psychosocial services in cancer care in the United States. Psycho-Oncology. 2013;22(3):699–703.
3. Nekhlyudov L, Ganz PA, Arora NK, Rowland JH. Going beyond being lost in transition: a decade of progress in cancer survivorship. J Clin Oncol. 2017;35(18):1978–81.

4. Sanft T, Denlinger CS, Armenian S, et al. NCCN guidelines insights: survivorship, version 2.2019. J Natl Compr Cancer Netw. 2019;17(7):784–94.
5. Riba MB, Donovan KA, Andersen B, et al. Distress management, version 3.2019, NCCN clinical practice guidelines in oncology. J Natl Compr Cancer Netw. 2019;17(10):1229–49.
6. Ploos van Amstel FK, van den Berg SW, van Laarhoven HW, Gielissen MF, Prins JB, Ottevanger PB. Distress screening remains important during follow-up after primary breast cancer treatment. Support Care Cancer. 2013;21(8):2107–15.
7. Roerink SH, de Ridder M, Prins J, et al. High level of distress in long-term survivors of thyroid carcinoma: results of rapid screening using the distress thermometer. Acta oncologica (Stockholm, Sweden). 2013;52(1):128–37.
8. Carmack CL, Basen-Engquist K, Gritz ER. Survivors at higher risk for adverse late outcomes due to psychosocial and behavioral risk factors. Cancer Epidemiol Biomark Preven: a publication of the American Association for Cancer Research, cosponsored by the American Society of Preventive Oncology. 2011;20(10):2068–77.
9. Swartzman S, Booth JN, Munro A, Sani F. Posttraumatic stress disorder after cancer diagnosis in adults: a meta-analysis. Depress Anxiety. 2017;34(4):327–39.
10. Brown JC, Huedo-Medina TB, Pescatello LS, et al. The efficacy of exercise in reducing depressive symptoms among cancer survivors: a meta-analysis. PLoS One. 2012;7(1):e30955.
11. Zhu G, Zhang X, Wang Y, Xiong H, Zhao Y, Sun F. Effects of exercise intervention in breast cancer survivors: a meta-analysis of 33 randomized controlled trails. Onco Targets Ther. 2016;9:2153–68.
12. Mendes DD, Mello MF, Ventura P, Passarela Cde M, Mari JJ. A systematic review on the effectiveness of cognitive behavioral therapy for posttraumatic stress disorder. Int J Psychiatry Med. 2008;38(3):241–59.
13. Lengacher CA, Reich RR, Paterson CL, et al. Examination of broad symptom improvement resulting from mindfulness-based stress reduction in breast cancer survivors: a randomized controlled trial. J Clin Oncol. 2016;34(24):2827–34.
14. Bower JE, Crosswell AD, Stanton AL, et al. Mindfulness meditation for younger breast cancer survivors: a randomized controlled trial. Cancer. 2015;121(8):1231–40.
15. Carlson LE, Doll R, Stephen J, et al. Randomized controlled trial of mindfulness-based cancer recovery versus supportive expressive group therapy for distressed survivors of breast cancer. J Clin Oncol. 2013;31(25):3119–26.
16. Carlson LE, Tamagawa R, Stephen J, Drysdale E, Zhong L, Speca M. Randomized-controlled trial of mindfulness-based cancer recovery versus supportive expressive group therapy among distressed breast cancer survivors (MINDSET): long-term follow-up results. Psycho-Oncology. 2016;25(7):750–9.
17. Bower JE. Cancer-related fatigue--mechanisms, risk factors, and treatments. Nat Rev Clin Oncol. 2014;11(10):597–609.
18. Husson O, Mols F, van de Poll-Franse L, de Vries J, Schep G, Thong MS. Variation in fatigue among 6011 (long-term) cancer survivors and a normative population: a study from the population-based PROFILES registry. Support Care Cancer. 2015;23(7):2165–74.
19. Mendoza TR, Wang XS, Cleeland CS, et al. The rapid assessment of fatigue severity in cancer patients: use of the Brief Fatigue Inventory. Cancer. 1999;85(5):1186–96.
20. de Raaf PJ, de Klerk C, Timman R, Busschbach JJ, Oldenmenger WH, van der Rijt CC. Systematic monitoring and treatment of physical symptoms to alleviate fatigue in patients with advanced cancer: a randomized controlled trial. J Clin Oncol. 2013;31(6):716–23.
21. Cramp F, Byron-Daniel J. Exercise for the management of cancer-related fatigue in adults. Cochrane Database Syst Rev. 2012;11:Cd006145.
22. Mustian KM, Alfano CM, Heckler C, et al. Comparison of pharmaceutical, psychological, and exercise treatments for cancer-related fatigue: a meta-analysis. JAMA Oncol. 2017;3(7):961–8.
23. Duijts SF, Faber MM, Oldenburg HS, van Beurden M, Aaronson NK. Effectiveness of behavioral techniques and physical exercise on psychosocial functioning and health-related

quality of life in breast cancer patients and survivors--a meta-analysis. Psycho-Oncology. 2011;20(2):115–26.
24. Posadzki P, Moon TW, Choi TY, Park TY, Lee MS, Ernst E. Acupuncture for cancer-related fatigue: a systematic review of randomized clinical trials. Support Care Cancer. 2013;21(7):2067–73.
25. Zeng Y, Luo T, Finnegan-John J, Cheng AS. Meta-analysis of randomized controlled trials of acupuncture for cancer-related fatigue. Integr Cancer Ther. 2014;13(3):193–200.
26. Pachman DR, Barton DL, Swetz KM, Loprinzi CL. Troublesome symptoms in cancer survivors: fatigue, insomnia, neuropathy, and pain. J Clin Oncol. 2012;30(30):3687–96.
27. Johannsen M, O'Connor M, O'Toole MS, Jensen AB, Hojris I, Zachariae R. Efficacy of mindfulness-based cognitive therapy on late post-treatment pain in women treated for primary breast cancer: a randomized controlled trial. J Clin Oncol. 2016;34(28):3390–9.
28. Huang ST, Good M, Zauszniewski JA. The effectiveness of music in relieving pain in cancer patients: a randomized controlled trial. Int J Nurs Stud. 2010;47(11):1354–62.
29. Cassileth DR, Keefe FJ. Integrative and behavioral approaches to the treatment of cancer-related neuropathic pain. Oncologist. 2010;15(Suppl 2):19–23.
30. Kwekkeboom KL, Cherwin CH, Lee JW, Wanta B. Mind-body treatments for the pain-fatigue-sleep disturbance symptom cluster in persons with cancer. J Pain Symptom Manag. 2010;39(1):126–38.
31. Irwin ML, Cartmel B, Gross CP, et al. Randomized exercise trial of aromatase inhibitor-induced arthralgia in breast cancer survivors. J Clin Oncol. 2015;33(10):1104–11.
32. Peppone LJ, Janelsins MC, Kamen C, et al. The effect of YOCAS(c)(R) yoga for musculoskeletal symptoms among breast cancer survivors on hormonal therapy. Breast Cancer Res Treat. 2015;150(3):597–604.
33. Ahles TA, Saykin AJ, McDonald BC, et al. Longitudinal assessment of cognitive changes associated with adjuvant treatment for breast cancer: impact of age and cognitive reserve. J Clin Oncol. 2010;28(29):4434–40.
34. Schmidt JE, Beckjord E, Bovbjerg DH, et al. Prevalence of perceived cognitive dysfunction in survivors of a wide range of cancers: results from the 2010 LIVESTRONG survey. J Cancer Survivorship Res Pract. 2016;10(2):302–11.
35. Ferguson RJ, McDonald BC, Rocque MA, et al. Development of CBT for chemotherapy-related cognitive change: results of a waitlist control trial. Psycho-Oncology. 2012;21(2):176–86.
36. Ferguson RJ, Sigmon ST, Pritchard AJ, et al. A randomized trial of videoconference-delivered cognitive behavioral therapy for survivors of breast cancer with self-reported cognitive dysfunction. Cancer. 2016;122(11):1782–91.
37. Hartman SJ, Nelson SH, Myers E, et al. Randomized controlled trial of increasing physical activity on objectively measured and self-reported cognitive functioning among breast cancer survivors: the memory & motion study. Cancer. 2018;124(1):192–202.
38. Chan RJ, McCarthy AL, Devenish J, Sullivan KA, Chan A. Systematic review of pharmacologic and non-pharmacologic interventions to manage cognitive alterations after chemotherapy for breast cancer. Eur J Cancer (Oxford, England : 1990). 2015;51(4):437–50.
39. Johns SA, Von Ah D, Brown LF, et al. Randomized controlled pilot trial of mindfulness-based stress reduction for breast and colorectal cancer survivors: effects on cancer-related cognitive impairment. J Cancer Survivorship Res Pract. 2016;10(3):437–48.
40. Derry HM, Jaremka LM, Bennett JM, et al. Yoga and self-reported cognitive problems in breast cancer survivors: a randomized controlled trial. Psycho-Oncology. 2015;24(8):958–66.
41. Campbell PT, Patel AV, Newton CC, Jacobs EJ, Gapstur SM. Associations of recreational physical activity and leisure time spent sitting with colorectal cancer survival. J Clin Oncol. 2013;31(7):876–85.
42. Kabat GC, Matthews CE, Kamensky V, Hollenbeck AR, Rohan TE. Adherence to cancer prevention guidelines and cancer incidence, cancer mortality, and total mortality: a prospective cohort study. Am J Clin Nutr. 2015;101(3):558–69.

43. Van Blarigan EL, Fuchs CS, Niedzwiecki D, et al. Association of survival with adherence to the American Cancer Society nutrition and physical activity guidelines for cancer survivors after colon cancer diagnosis: the CALGB 89803/Alliance trial. JAMA Oncol. 2018;4(6):783–90.
44. Jones LW, Liu Q, Armstrong GT, et al. Exercise and risk of major cardiovascular events in adult survivors of childhood hodgkin lymphoma: a report from the childhood cancer survivor study. J Clin Oncol. 2014;32(32):3643–50.
45. Jones LW, Habel LA, Weltzien E, et al. Exercise and risk of cardiovascular events in women with nonmetastatic breast cancer. J Clin Oncol. 2016;34(23):2743–9.
46. Blaney JM, Lowe-Strong A, Rankin-Watt J, Campbell A, Gracey JH. Cancer survivors' exercise barriers, facilitators and preferences in the context of fatigue, quality of life and physical activity participation: a questionnaire-survey. Psycho-Oncology. 2013;22(1):186–94.
47. Demark-Wahnefried W, Clipp EC, Lipkus IM, et al. Main outcomes of the FRESH START trial: a sequentially tailored, diet and exercise mailed print intervention among breast and prostate cancer survivors. J Clin Oncol. 2007;25(19):2709–18.
48. Halpern MT, Viswanathan M, Evans TS, Birken SA, Basch E, Mayer DK. Models of cancer survivorship care: overview and summary of current evidence. J Oncol Pract. 2015;11(1):e19–27.
49. Wattchow DA, Weller DP, Esterman A, et al. General practice vs surgical-based follow-up for patients with colon cancer: randomised controlled trial. Br J Cancer. 2006;94(8):1116–21.
50. Grunfeld E, Levine MN, Julian JA, et al. Randomized trial of long-term follow-up for early-stage breast cancer: a comparison of family physician versus specialist care. J Clin Oncol. 2006;24(6):848–55.
51. Mani S, Khera N, Rybicki L, et al. Primary care physician perspectives on caring for adult survivors of hematologic malignancies and hematopoietic cell transplantation. Clin Lymphoma Myeloma Leuk. 2020;20(2):70–7.
52. Kokko R, Hakama M, Holli K. Follow-up cost of breast cancer patients with localized disease after primary treatment: a randomized trial. Breast Cancer Res Treat. 2005;93(3):255–60.
53. Jacobsen PB, DeRosa AP, Henderson TO, et al. Systematic review of the impact of cancer survivorship care plans on health outcomes and health care delivery. J Clin Oncol. 2018;36(20):2088–100.
54. Chubak J, Tuzzio L, Hsu C, et al. Providing care for cancer survivors in integrated health care delivery systems: practices, challenges, and research opportunities. J Oncol Pract. 2012;8(3):184–9.
55. Ferraro CS, Bernhard L, Coffman J, Majhail NS, Hamilton BK. Optimizing long-term Care for Hematopoietic Cell Transplantation (HCT) survivors: framework for establishing a new Blood and Marrow Transplant (BMT) survivorship program. Biol Blood Marrow Transplant. 2018;24(3):S266.
56. Nonzee NJ, Ragas DM, Ha Luu T, et al. Delays in Cancer care among low-income minorities despite access. J Womens Health (Larchmt). 2015;24(6):506–14.

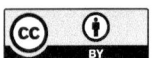

Chapter 12
Starting a Palliative Care Program at a Cancer Center

Laura Shoemaker and Susan McInnes

Background

While previously a resource only found in large academic hospitals or specialized community-based healthcare agencies, palliative care (PC) has become an essential part of modern health care in the United States (US) and around the world. A status report in the Journal of Palliative Medicine in 2016 reported that 67% of US hospitals with 50 or more total facility beds and 90% of hospitals with 300 beds or more reported the presence of a palliative care program [1]. The presence of inpatient PC programs varied regionally, with the highest percentage in the Northeast and the lowest in the South [1]. Outpatient access to PC has also grown, both in the clinic setting and in the community [2, 3]. As clinical access has grown, so has the body of evidence about the positive impact of PC. A wide range of data demonstrates the important role PC plays in care quality, patient and family satisfaction, clinician experience, and healthcare resource utilization [4–7]. Alignment with this "quadruple aim" positions PC to be a key player in future healthcare transformation and the movement toward value-based care [8].

The Center to Advance Palliative Care (CAPC) defines "palliative care" as specialized medical care for people living with a serious illness. The term was coined in 1974 by Dr. Balfour Mount, a surgical oncologist at The Royal Victoria Hospital of McGill University in Montreal, Canada. Mount likely created the new term to circumvent existing negative connotations many had with hospice. Dame Cicely Saunders, considered the founder of both the modern hospice movement and the field of PC, developed and propagated the clinical practice around her concept of "Total Pain." Total Pain refers to the comprehensive, multifaceted experience of suffering associated with serious illness, which Saunders further divided into four

L. Shoemaker (✉) · S. McInnes
Department of Palliative & Supportive Care, Taussig Cancer Institute, Cleveland Clinic, Cleveland, OH, USA
e-mail: shoemal@ccf.org; mcinnes@ccf.org

M. Aljurf et al. (eds.), *The Comprehensive Cancer Center*,
https://doi.org/10.1007/978-3-030-82052-7_12

domains: physical, emotional, social, and spiritual [9]. A commitment to improve quality of life by attending to all of these dimensions of suffering remains central to the practice of PC today. Consistent with this comprehensive approach, interdisciplinary team-based care by physicians, nurses (including advance practice nurses), social workers, chaplains, and complementary therapists is fundamental. PC is appropriate at any age and at any stage in a serious illness and is provided along with curative treatment. Thus, the provision of PC is based on the needs of the patient, not on the patient's prognosis.

Palliative care has played a central role in the delivery of high-quality cancer care for some time, likely stemming from the fact that many of the early PC practitioners were oncologists. While specialty PC practice and training has grown to encompass serious illnesses of all types, PC remains heavily focused on supportive cancer care. The National Comprehensive Cancer Network (NCCN) guidelines direct: "institutions should develop processes for integrating palliative care into cancer care, both as part of usual oncology care and for patients with specialty palliative care needs." [10] A wide body of evidence has demonstrated PC's impact on cancer care quality throughout the trajectory of cancer care in a wide variety of malignancies and care settings [11–14]. In addition to addressing the aim to palliate symptoms, systematic early integration of PC has shown to prolong survival [15]. Consistent with PC's aim to facilitate individualized, patient-centered plans of care, research has demonstrated that those who receive PC consultations have care plans aligned with their goals and care that costs less overall [6, 16, 17]. As a result, PC metrics have been incorporated into cancer-focused, value-based care approaches, like the Center for Medicare and Medicaid's Advanced Alternative Payment Model, the Oncology Care Model (https://innovation.cms.gov/innovation-models/oncology-care).

Although specialty PC has become an integral part of high-quality cancer care, PC services are not ubiquitous, and access to PC is still limited in many areas and care settings. The reasons for limited access vary by locale and include specialty PC workforce constraints, lack of financial support for PC staffing resources, and variable engagement by clinicians and healthcare leadership. Despite these challenges, many healthcare professionals and institutions remain committed to establishing new specialty PC service lines, a complex but worthwhile endeavor. The following sections of this chapter will focus on the steps and anticipated challenges in initiating and integrating specialty PC within a cancer care entity. The stages have been broken into Planning (early and late), Launch and Integration, and Monitoring and Sustainability.

Planning

Early Planning

The first step in starting a new PC service line is engaging PC champions and institutional leadership. Quite often, new PC programs or service lines are created in response to requests, or even, demands from existing clinicians (physicians, nurses, care managers). Engaging these frontline allies simultaneously as one petitions institutional leadership for financial support can be effective in generating support for the initiation of a new PC service line. Fortunately, "making the [financial] case" for the integration of PC in cancer care is no longer a difficult task. As described above, a wide variety of evidence exists to support PC's role in supporting outcomes around care quality, patient/provider satisfaction, and healthcare utilization. These published outcomes can be complemented by analysis of local data, including:

- Clinical volumes by cancer diagnosis.
- Acute admissions and/or ED visits.
- Hospital and/or ICU length of stay (LOS).
- Hospice utilization (referral rates and LOS on hospice).
- Prevalence of moderate to severe symptoms.
- Rate of advance directive completion.

Subjective reports from patients, families, and providers about care gaps can also be compelling data when advocating for resource allocation to a new PC service line. As organizational leadership is engaged, it is essential to understand and then align PC service line goals with those of the larger institution.

Once conceptual alignment between organizational and PC leadership is achieved, early planning should also include a focused "needs assessment" to identify what the patients, families, clinicians, and institution want and need most from a specialty PC team. There are a wide variety of reasons to start PC programs, and no inaugural program can address all possible needs from the start. Building comprehensive PC programs across care settings takes years to decades. When starting a new PC program, it is important to identify focused, key aims that address high-priority patient care or provider practice needs. The following list represents only a few of the many possible "needs" for initiating a new PC service:

- Management of complex, time-consuming cancer-related pain, especially in the setting of increasing regulatory requirements around opioid prescribing.
- Underutilization of hospice care, including low rates referrals and/or short length of stay on hospice care.
- High-level psychosocial distress in patients in families around coping with the challenges of cancer care.
- Facilitation of conversations around care goals and preferences in patients with long hospital length of stay or those ideintified as "high utilizers" of healthcare resources.

Designing the PC service line according to the most pressing needs will increase the likelihood of successful achievement of shared goals. Once there is alignment around focused goals, shared outcome measures can be created. Clearly outlining the anticipated "deliverables" is an important next step in considering the design of a new PC service line. Typical deliverables include clinical symptom management (pain and non-pain symptoms), facilitation of discussions about patient care goals and preferences, transitions from disease-directed therapy to comfort-focused care, the provision of comfort focused and end-of-life care, psychosocial support, spiritual support, and complementary therapies like music, art, Reiki, meditation. An effective PC service does not need to include all components listed here in order to be successful, especially at the start of the service. On the contrary, PC services that are built piece by piece, starting where needs and engagement are highest, are most likely to be successful. Teams or institutions who try to tackle every PC need, everywhere (outpatient, inpatient, and in the community) all at once may be quickly overrun by unmanageable referral volumes, unmet expectations, and strained clinical teams. Depending on available resources and primary aims, goals can further be tailored to a specific malignancy or stage (e.g., allogeneic stem cell transplantation or metastatic lung cancer). The importance of the early planning stage, including engagement of institutional leadership and alignment around shared goals, cannot be underestimated. The Center to Advance Palliative Care has a robust collection of materials available online for members for PC program planning, design, and execution (www.CAPC.org).

Late Planning

Once primary objectives and outcomes have been established, the next step is designing the PC service line, with consideration to care setting and staffing scheme. While staffing models may ultimately be limited by resource allocation, it is important to design a service line that will address the primary objectives. For example, if the primary objective is complex pain and symptom management in patients with advanced solid tumors, starting an outpatient PC service with an experienced physician embedded within the outpatient oncology clinic would be an advisable first step. If the primary need is symptom management during an admission for an allogeneic stem cell transplant, then embedding a PC clinician (either physician or advance practice provider (APP, includes nurse practitioner or physician assistant)) on the transplant unit may be more appropriate. If the resources and request for PC are coming from hospital leadership, the needs may be centered on ICU throughput, hospital length of stay, or inpatient readmissions. In this case, a consultative interdisciplinary inpatient PC team to help facilitate conversations around care goals and preferences may be the right place to start. Alternatively, if the resources and engagement are from an institutional or community-based hospice organization with an aim to increase timely referrals and offer earlier service to high-risk patients in the community, it may make sense to start with an interdisciplinary community-based PC team to capture referrals upon hospital discharge or via insurance claims-based data. Table 12.1 outlines the primary PC delivery models and the associated target outcomes, team composition, and support needs. These PC delivery models can include:

- Inpatient consultation.
- Inpatient primary admitting service, with or without a designated physical space or unit.

Table 12.1 Palliative care delivery models

Service type	Target outcomes	Team clinicians	Support needs
Inpatient consultation	Hospital-based metrics like hospital or ICU LOS or readmissions Facilitation of discussion about care goals and preferences Transitions from disease-directed plan of care to comfort-focused plan of care Symptom management	Physician and/or APP Social work Spiritual care	Team office space Administrative practice management
Inpatient admitting	Consultative needs as above Desire to "hand-off" PC patients from medical, surgical and ICU services Physical space to attend to the care of actively dying patients	Physician APP (per service volumes) Social work Spiritual care Dedicated RN workforce Care manager Hospice liaison	Inpatient space/unit Team office space Administrative practice management Alignment with institutional or collaborating hospice agency
Outpatient clinic	Symptom management Support for conversations regarding care goals and preferences Disease or malignancy specific integration	Physician or APP RN care coordinator Social work (if not already available within cancer center)	Clinic space Scheduling staff Staff for patient check-in and rooming Administrative practice management
Community-based	Facilitation of discussion about care goals and preferences Transitions from disease-directed plan of care to comfort-focused plan of care Symptom management Acute care utilization metrics[a]	Physician or APP Social work Spiritual care RN care coordinator	Team office space Scheduling staff Administrative practice management

[a]The ability to impact acute care utilization metrics depends on the design of a community-based PC program

- Outpatient clinic, either embedded within a target specialty or stand-alone.
- Community-based, offering visits to patients in home and facilities, in person or virtually.

The decision about staffing the service with a physician or an APP depends on a number of factors including clinical acuity, healthcare system culture, and available workforce. A team that includes *both* a physician and an APP supports both the interdisciplinary practice of PC and facilitates management of higher clinical volumes.

Decisions should be made early about what kind of symptoms and which patient populations the PC team will manage. For example, will an inpatient PC team's services be available to all patients, only patients with an identifiable serious illness, patients in the ICU or RNF, or focused on particular diagnoses like cancer? This is especially important when considering pain management, which can quickly consume staffing resources. Will the team manage cancer pain, pain related to serious illness, chronic pain, postsurgical pain, complex or refractory pain syndromes?

Once a commitment has been made about resource allocation, care delivery setting, and staffing scheme, it is time to plan the implementation of the PC service by establishing a timeline. Due to specialty PC workforce constraints and training needs, recruitment is often the limiting step in service initiation. In the United States, it may take 6–24 months to recruit a fellowship-trained PC physician. APP staffing is often available within a much shorter time frame; however, many APP recruits do not have specialty PC training or experience. Therefore, a 6–12 month period for training must be allowed. For institutions who do not have existing PC specialists, it is advisable to start with an experienced or fellowship-trained PC physician. This provider will come equipped to deliver specialty PC from the start of their employment and may serve as a resource to train APP hires as the service grows. CAPC has extensive online training resources to support the development of the entire interdisciplinary team. PC certification pathways (available for physicians, nurse practitioners, social workers, and chaplains) offer additional opportunities for professional development of the PC team.

If not already in existence (and engaged with planning the service line), an administrative team should be assembled after the clinical team is recruited. The administrative team can support service integration by identifying team space, coordinating credentialing, reviewing pertinent hospital bylaws and standard operating procedures, and setting up meetings with potential referral sources and PC service champions. Furthermore, developing an integration "Steering Committee" composed of the institutions' PC champions, healthcare system leadership, and other key stakeholders will help facilitate a successful launch. Typical steering committee members include leadership, chief nursing officers, finance, marketing and communications, pharmacy, spiritual care, and complementary care services.

Prior to service launch, it is important to clarify operational standards around service hours, evening on call and weekend coverage, the time frame within which to see new referrals, follow-up frequency and duration, and communication processes for referral sources and other bedside caregivers. Routine team workflows, such as clinical huddles and interdisciplinary team meetings, can then be designed to support these expectations and facilitate effective communication within the PC team.

Launch and Integration

Despite the wider access to and presence of PC, many healthcare professionals and lay public still lack an understanding of what PC encompasses. PC is often confused with hospice or end-of-life care, such that physicians who refer to PC sometimes have trouble articulating to patients why they are making the referral and what outcomes to expect from the referral. Simply put, palliative care is specialized medical care for people living with a serious illness. The ultimate goal is to improve quality of life for both the patient and the family, which is often achieved through palliation of symptoms and enhanced communication with patients and families about their care preferences, goals, and plans. While end-of-life care is a critical part of PC, it is only a part of what PC envelops. Addressing this knowledge deficit about PC is essential when launching a new specialty PC service. In addition to clearly communicating what PC is, it is helpful to share simple, concise language (e.g., an "elevator speech") for referring clinicians, healthcare leadership, and other PC champions to use when interacting with patients and other healthcare professionals.

At or just prior to service launch, one should organize meetings or schedule presentations for stakeholders, like institutional leadership, shared governance teams, medical and nursing staff, medical educators, and care management. These engagements serve several functions by creating a forum to: (1) address the existing gaps in understanding about what PC is, (2) set expectations about what this new service line will deliver, and (3) clarify referral processes. Attendees need to leave these presentations understanding: (1) who may place referrals (is referral limited to physicians or can other clinicians refer?), (2) why to refer a patient (what are the clinical eligibility criteria?), (3) when to refer a patient (either during a hospital stay or along their trajectory of serious illness), and (4) how to communicate a new patient referral to the patient and PC team (electronic, telephone, etc.).

A successful service line launch is ultimately dependent on the development of meaningful relationships between the PC team and other clinicians within the care setting. Intentional steps to enhance visibility, like presence in clinical care areas, participation with hospital or clinic committees, and supporting educational or training efforts go a long way in helping establish the PC team. Prioritizing thoughtful, effective communication with referring providers and other bedside clinicians also helps develop trust and service line success.

Monitoring and Sustainability

Monitoring the activities of the PC service entails collecting data from a number of sources. An "Advisory Committee," composed of stakeholders and high utilizers of the service can be a key source of information. While this committee may include some of the participants from the Steering Committee, it can envelop a larger scope to include key referral sources, such as large medical or specialty practices, ICU clinicians, and patient/family councils. The goal is to get real-time input from end users for early identification of best practices, service gaps, or emerging challenges. The PC team itself will be another great source of data. Scheduling regular team meetings with the aim of collecting experiential feedback supplements standard data points like clinical volumes, service outcomes, and patient/family experience scores. PC team meetings also create a forum for team members to share successes and best practices and collaborate around challenges in care delivery.

Successful integration of the PC service is often marked by increasing referral volumes over time. Developing thresholds for hiring additional staff supports ongoing incremental growth. Understanding the reasons for referral, the average number of visits per referral, and the referral sources themselves will direct what kind of additional staff is needed. Often, PC team bandwidth can be expanded by adding interdisciplinary clinicians like APPs, social workers, chaplains, and care coordinators. If the service is started in one care setting (inpatient or outpatient), the next step for expansion may be a complementary PC service in the alternate setting. Building a comprehensive PC program with clinical services available in a variety of care settings ultimately creates a continuum of support to follow a patient across care transitions and throughout the trajectory of a serious illness. When considering the most advanced stages of a serious illness, it is important to either provide hospice care (or similar end-of-life care) or partner closely with a high-quality hospice organization. This will assure that patients and families receive optional care throughout the duration of their illness.

Quality

The availability of PC services is essential to quality cancer care. Organizations such as the Multinational Agency for Supportive Care in Cancer (MASCC), American Society for Clinical Oncology (ASCO), the NCCN, and the American College of Surgeons Commission on Cancer (CoC) have issued guidelines and standards for the provision of PC services to cancer patients from early in the course of illness, throughout the disease course and at end of life [10, 16, 18, 19]. ASCO had also issued guidelines for PC in the global setting, stratified by resource availability [20]. This guideline outlines quality PC for patients with cancer in resource-constrained settings under various models of care. Consistent among all guidelines and standards are recommendations and/or requirements including the following:

- Interdisciplinary care is essential to identify and address physical, psychological, spiritual, social, and cultural aspects of care.
- PC services are ideally available on-site at a cancer center but may also be provided by referral to care partners in the community.
- PC begins at diagnosis and may be initially provided by the oncology team (primary palliative care) with availability of specialist palliative care team consultation.
- Quality PC should be provided in accordance with established evidence-based national and international guidelines.

The most robust recently updated guidelines were developed as a national consensus project among 13 member organizations and are summarized in Table 12.2 [21].

Table 12.2 Guidelines for quality palliative care

Domain	Guideline
Structure and process of care	Interdisciplinary team (IDT)
	Comprehensive palliative care assessment
	Palliative care plan
	Continuity of palliative care
	Care settings
	IDT education
	Coordination of care and care transitions
	Emotional support to the IDT
	Continuous quality improvement
	Stability, sustainability, and growth
Physical aspects of care	Global
	Screening and assessment
	Treatment
	Ongoing care
Psychological and psychiatric aspects of care	Global
	Screening and assessment
	Treatment
	Ongoing care
Social aspects of care	Global
	Screening and assessment
	Treatment
	Ongoing care
Spiritual, religious, and existential aspects of care	Global
	Screening and assessment
	Treatment
	Ongoing care
Cultural aspects of care	Global
	Communication and language
	Screening and assessment
	Treatment
Care of the patient nearing end of life	Interdisciplinary team
	Screening and assessment
	Treatment before death
	Treatment during the dying process and immediately after death
	Bereavement
Ethical and legal aspects of care	Global
	Legal considerations
	Screening and assessment
	Treatment and ongoing decision-making

Table adapted from: Ferrell et al. [21]

Palliative care programs have many resources available to help determine how to assess and improve quality of their care. Palliative provider education is integral to quality care, and palliative certification ensures a strong knowledge base for the interdisciplinary team, including physicians, advance practice providers, nurses, social workers, and chaplains. There are abundant online opportunities for ongoing education through the American Academy for Hospice and Palliative Medicine (www.AAHPM.org), the Center to Advance Palliative Care (www.capc.org), MASCC (https://www.mascc.org/palliative-care), and the World Health Organization (https://www.who.int/cancer/palliative/en/).

As a palliative program is developed, it is critical to include evaluation of the structure, process and outcomes of the program from the outset. This ensures that the best care is provided to those who need it most. Importantly, ongoing evaluation identifies best practices and opportunities for ongoing quality improvement initiatives. Recently, several national quality registries in the United States have been merged to become the Palliative Care Quality Collaborative and plan to establish the Palliative Care Quality Initiative (PCQC), a registry anticipated to open in 2021 to capture both patient and program quality data.

Metrics specific to palliative care have been proposed by AAHPM in the Measuring What Matters project [22]. The top ten metrics are: comprehensive assessment, screening for physical symptoms, pain treatment, dyspnea screening and management, discussion of emotional or psychological needs, discussion of spiritual/religious concerns, documentation of surrogate, treatment preferences, care consistency with documented care preferences, and a global measure such as quality of life [23]. CAPC has published updated suggested quality metrics which is shown in Table 12.3 [24]. Key illustrations of patient quality are access to palliative care, pain assessment and management, safe opioid prescribing practices, and documentation of advance directives (ADs). Program quality measures may include patient satisfaction scores, hospital readmission rate, ICU utilization near end of life, and days on hospice care. Palliative programs can select areas they wish to prioritize based on their care delivery models.

Ongoing continuous improvement is the mainstay of quality care. In fact, a focus on improving quality is intrinsic to the patient-centered discipline of palliative care [25]. Tracking quality metrics allows for rapid recognition of areas a program can improve care. Quality improvement (QI) projects can then be tailored to improving care in a specific area such as AD completion rates or accurate, safe opioid prescribing. QI projects are best accomplished by a multidisciplinary team of engaged stakeholders who wish to facilitate sustainable change. Basic QI methodology includes identification of a problem to be addressed, measuring and defining goals, root cause analysis, rapid cycle plan-do-study-act interventions and plans for sustainability and spread. The Institute for Healthcare Improvement Open School initiative offers free courses in QI methodology to support programs wishing to learn a model for improvement (www.ihi.org).

Table 12.3 Quality measures recommended by the Center to Advance Palliative Care [24]

Measure category	Measure type	Measure/measure area
Access	Structure	Availability of interdisciplinary palliative care team, with 24/7 response of some kind in selected facility(ies)
Satisfaction	Patient experience	Consumer assessment of health providers and systems (CAHPS)
Satisfaction	Outcome	Likelihood to recommend the services or program (i.e., net promoter score)
Advance care planning	Process	Rates of patients who have an advance care plan or surrogate decision maker documented in the medical record or documentation in the medical record that an advance care plan was discussed but the patient did not wish or was not able to name a surrogate decision maker or provide an advance care plan
Clinical quality	Process	Proportion of patients with pain screening or assessment (and/or with pain plan of care)
Clinical quality	Process	Proportion of patients with functional assessment (ability to perform activities of daily living and instrumental activities of daily living)
Clinical quality	Process	Proportion of patients with their caregiver burden formally assessed
Utilization	Outcome	Rates of avoidable hospital and/or emergency department utilization; risk-adjusted as appropriate
Utilization	Outcome	Days at home: Number of days a patient remains outside of an institutional care setting during a standardized time period
Utilization	Process	Appropriate hospice utilization (e.g., hospice referral rate or hospice length of stay (LOS) for those referred or proportion of hospice LOS less than 7 days or more than 180 days for those referred)

Additional details and resources are available at https://www.capc.org/defining-and-measuring-quality/

Research

Establishing a research framework is foundational to developing and sustaining palliative care services. The concept of research begins with asking questions and discovering new knowledge to help better care for our patients. Creating a database of patients for QI purposes at the outset allows for evaluation of quality and can also help identify areas for future research in symptom management, novel care delivery models, and palliative care education. Such a database should incorporate assessments, measurements, and outcomes. Any new research protocol would need to be approved by an institutional review board (IRB), which may be on-site or affiliated.

Palliative care research has expanded significantly over the past decade. Competitive funding sources support well-designed palliative clinical trials that are published in high-impact journals and result in practice-changing outcomes. A prime example of this is the randomized trial of early palliative care for outpatients with metastatic non-small cell lung cancer [15]. Patients who received early specialist palliative care had better quality of life, less depressive symptoms, less aggressive end-of-life care, and longer median survival that those with usual care. Now early palliative care for such patients is recognized as the standard of care and a best practice. More recent examples are the randomized trials of integration of palliative care into the care of patients undergoing hematopoietic stem cell transplantation and acute myeloid leukemia induction, affirming better quality of life and less anxiety for those who received palliative care [26–28].

In order for research to have impact, findings must be shared. There are multiple venues to share QI and clinical trial results. AAHPM, CAPC, National Hospice and Palliative Care Organization (NHPCO), ASCO, and IHI have annual assemblies with opportunities to present posters and oral abstracts. In additional, McGill University in Montreal, Canada, offers a long-running International Congress on Palliative Care with written and oral presentations. In addition, there are many palliative journals dedicated to palliative research, and cancer-specific journals such as *Journal of Clinical Oncology* (JCO), *JCO Oncology Practice*, *JAMA Oncology*, and others which also publish impactful palliative oncology research.

Conclusion

Palliative care, focused on the optimization of quality of life, has become an essential part of cancer care. While the prevalence of PC has grown, access is still limited in a variety of care settings, institutions, and geographic locations. Developing and launching a specialty PC service enhances cancer care and helps address unmet needs related to cancer symptoms, communication about care goals and preferences, and transitions in care. Planning for the integration of a new palliative care service is a complex process that requires attention to thorough planning, as well as attentive execution and monitoring to assure delivery of sustainable, interdisciplinary, and high-quality care. Cancer centers need to strategically invest in this area as they progress towards provision of comprehensive cancer care services to patients.

References

1. Dumanovsky T, Augustin R, Rogers M, Lettang K, Meier DE, Morrison RS. The growth of palliative care in U.S. hospitals: a status report. J Palliat Med. 2016;19(1):8–15.
2. Rabow M, Kvale E, Barbour L, et al. Moving upstream: a review of the evidence of the impact of outpatient palliative care. J Palliat Med. 2013;16(12):1540–9.

3. Gibson S, Bordofsky M, Hirsch J, Kearney M, Solis M, Wong C. Community palliative care: one community's experience providing outpatient palliative care. J Hosp Palliat Nurs. 2012;14(7):491–9.
4. Enguidanos S, Vesper E, Lorenz K. 30-day readmissions among seriously ill older adults. J Palliat Med. 2012;15(12):1356–61.
5. Kerr CW, Donohue KA, Tangeman JC, et al. Cost savings and enhanced hospice enrollment with a home-based palliative care program implemented as a hospice-private payer partnership. J Palliat Med. 2014;17(12):1328–35.
6. Morrison RS, Penrod JD, Cassel JB, et al. Cost savings associated with US hospital palliative care consultation programs. Arch Intern Med. 2008;168(16):1783–90.
7. O'Mahony S, Blank AE, Zallman L, Selwyn PA. The benefits of a hospital-based inpatient palliative care consultation service: preliminary outcome data. J Palliat Med. 2005;8(5):1033–9.
8. Bodenheimer T, Sinsky C. From triple to quadruple aim: care of the patient requires care of the provider. Ann Fam Med. 2014;12(6):573–6.
9. Clark D, Foley KM. Dame Cicely Saunders. The pharos of alpha omega alpha-honor medical society. Alpha Omega Alpha. 2003;66(3):8–10.
10. Dans M, Smith T, Back A, et al. NCCN guidelines insights: palliative care, version 2.2017. J Natl Compr Cancer Netw. 2017;15(8):989–97.
11. Jack B, Hillier V, Williams A, Oldham J. Hospital based palliative care teams improve the insight of cancer patients into their disease. Palliat Med. 2004;18(1):46–52.
12. Medicine Io. Dying in America: improving quality and honoring individual preferences near the end of life. Washington, DC: The National Academies Press; 2015.
13. Shoemaker LK, Estfan B, Induru R, Walsh TD. Symptom management: an important part of cancer care. Cleve Clin J Med. 2011;78(1):25–34.
14. Samala RV, Valent J, Noche N, Lagman R. Palliative care in patients with multiple myeloma. J Pain Symptom Manag. 2019;58(6):1113–8.
15. Temel JS, Greer JA, Muzikansky A, et al. Early palliative care for patients with metastatic non-small-cell lung cancer. N Engl J Med. 2010;363(8):733–42.
16. Ferrell BR, Temel JS, Temin S, et al. Integration of palliative care into standard oncology care: American Society of Clinical Oncology clinical practice guideline update. J Clin Oncol. 2017;35(1):96–112.
17. Smith TJ, Temin S, Alesi ER, et al. American Society of Clinical Oncology provisional clinical opinion: the integration of palliative care into standard oncology care. J Clin Oncol. 2012;30(8):880–7.
18. MASCC Guidelines. https://www.mascc.org/guidelines. Accessed 03/01/2021.
19. Commission on Cancer (CoC) Standards and Resources. https://www.facs.org/Quality-Programs/Cancer/CoC/standards. Accessed 03/01/2021.
20. Osman H, Shrestha S, Temin S, et al. Palliative Care in the Global Setting: ASCO resource-stratified practice guideline. J Glob Oncol. 2018;4:1–24.
21. Ferrell BR, Twaddle ML, Melnick A, Meier DE. National Consensus Project Clinical Practice Guidelines for quality palliative care guidelines, 4th edition. J Palliat Med. 2018;21(12):1684–9.
22. Dy SM, Kiley KB, Ast K, et al. Measuring what matters: top-ranked quality indicators for hospice and palliative care from the American Academy of Hospice and Palliative Medicine and Hospice and Palliative Nurses Association. J Pain Symptom Manag. 2015;49(4):773–81.
23. American Academy of Hospice and Palliative Medicine. Measuring What Matters. http://aahpm.org/quality/measuring-what-matters. Accessed 03/01/2021.
24. Center to Advance Palliative Care. Defining and measuring quality. https://www.capc.org/defining-and-measuring-quality/. Accessed 03/01/2021.
25. Kamal AH, Hanson LC, Casarett DJ, et al. The quality imperative for palliative care. J Pain Symptom Manag. 2015;49(2):243–53.

26. El-Jawahri A, LeBlanc T, VanDusen H, et al. Effect of inpatient palliative care on quality of life 2 weeks after hematopoietic stem cell transplantation: a randomized clinical trial. JAMA. 2016;316(20):2094–103.
27. El-Jawahri A, LeBlanc TW, Kavanaugh A, et al. Effectiveness of integrated palliative and oncology care for patients with acute myeloid leukemia: a randomized clinical trial. JAMA Oncol. 2021;7(2):238–45.
28. El-Jawahri A, Traeger L, Greer JA, et al. Effect of inpatient palliative care during hemato-poietic stem-cell transplant on psychological distress 6 months after transplant: results of a randomized clinical trial. J Clin Oncol. 2017;35(32):3714–21.

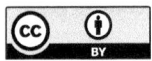

Chapter 13
Transplantation and Cellular Therapy

Navneet S. Majhail and Marcos De Lima

Introduction

Hematopoietic cell transplantation (HCT) is an established treatment for selected patients with high-risk hematologic malignancies and other malignant and non-malignant diseases. An estimated 50,000 transplantation procedures are performed worldwide annually [1]. The number of patients who need and receive HCT is expected to grow as transplantation becomes safer with advances in transplantation technology and supportive care, greater donor availability, emerging indications, and diffusion of this procedure to lower income and lower middle income countries. The increase in utilization of transplantation has been paralleled by improvement in outcomes, resulting in a larger number of transplant survivors who are potentially cured of their underlying disease [2–5]. Addressing the needs of long-term survivors is, therefore, a growing aspect of transplant programs. An added dimension to this is the advent of cellular therapies, especially chimeric antigen receptor (CAR) T-cell therapies, which are also included within the domain of transplantation programs. A comprehensive center should ideally consider provision of HCT procedures, both in the context of routine care and clinical trials. This chapter will review the foundational aspects required to establish a transplantation and cellular therapy program within an upcoming cancer center. The Worldwide Network for Blood and Marrow Transplantation (WBMT) has also published guidelines on establishing HCT program, with a specific focus on lower middle and lower income countries [6, 7].

N. S. Majhail (✉)
Blood and Marrow Transplant Program, Cleveland Clinic, Cleveland, OH, USA
e-mail: navneet.majhail@sarahcannon.com

M. De Lima
Blood and Marrow Transplant and Cellular Therapy, Ohio State University,
Columbus, OH, USA

Rationale for HCT and Cellular Therapy Program

HCT and cellular therapy are essential treatments as part of providing comprehensive care to cancer patients. There is a plethora of indications for transplantation, which mainly focus on hematologic malignancies [8, 9]. However, cancer centers will frequently manage patients with nonmalignant but life-threatening conditions that may warrant HCT (e.g., aplastic anemia). Furthermore, indications for transplantation in pediatric patients also include conditions such as inherited metabolic diseases and hemoglobinopathies that are treated with HCT. The expansion of cellular therapies and the emerging role of transplantation for autoimmune diseases is another area where an HCT program can serve a role in providing care for patients. Furthermore, an HCT program can serve as a resource for external referrals to a cancer center [10]. Overall, there continues to be a strong demand for the advanced treatment of patients with hematologic malignancies using HCT and cellular therapies [11, 12].

The need to have a dedicated resource in the form of an HCT program stems from the complexity of the procedure and its associated risks for severe morbidity and mortality, experience and expertise required of the team that manages patients, the logistical aspects around collection and ultimately infusion of hematopoietic progenitor cells, and the highly regulated nature of the procedure. Quality is an important component of care that is provided to patients, and international accreditation organizations such as the Foundation for the Accreditation of Cellular Therapies (FACT) and the Joint Accreditation for the International Society of Cellular Therapy and European Society for Blood and Marrow Transplantation (JACIE) provide minimum standards for a high-quality HCT program [13].

It needs to be recognized that in setting up an HCT program, investment in personnel and infrastructure is also needed for ancillary services that are critical to providing safe and high-quality care to HCT recipients. Some examples of these services include availability of blood bank support, specialized laboratory testing (e.g., for cytomegalovirus (CMV), infectious disease markers, pathology expertise), intensive care unit support, palliative care and hospice, and collaboration with experts in other specialties such as intensive care, nephrology etc. Patients also need a range of supportive care services, such as psychosocial and palliative care services, and local lodging for the patient and caregiver.

HCT Program Structure

Strong institutional commitment and support is needed before embarking on establishment of an HCT program, given the resources required and the expense involved. Planning for an HCT program requires a long-term vision and a phased approach, especially if the cancer center does not have experience with hematologic malignancies. Initial efforts need to be focused towards establishing a robust hematologic malignancy program, since they comprise the majority of indications for transplant, and many of the personnel competencies can be applied to the care of HCT recipients. As discussed below, establishment of ancillary support services should be planned in parallel to the plan for the HCT program. Prior to setting up a program for management of HCT recipients, it is prudent to dedicate resources and efforts to set up a robust hematologic malignancy program that gives clinicians and other staff the opportunity to obtain experience in managing patients with acute leukemia, lymphoma, and myeloma. Once the hematologic malignancy program has matured, a rational next step towards HCT is to begin with autologous transplantation, and then expand to human leukocyte antigen (HLA)-matched sibling donor allogeneic transplantation. Once sufficient experience has been obtained with these approaches, the program can expand to allogeneic transplantation using matched unrelated donors, haploidentical donors, and other alternative donor sources such as umbilical cord blood. Additionally, a new program may initially consider transplanting patients who are younger, have less comorbidities, and at lower risk for transplant-related complications. This phased approach gives the transplant team an opportunity to gain expertise as they evolve into the management of patients of increasing complexity, given that center volume and experience have been shown to be associated with outcomes [14, 15]. The availability of local resources that can collaborate or the ability to contract out certain services (e.g., apheresis through a local blood bank) may also be a factor in planning for the setup of a new program. Histocompatibility expertise is fundamental and may be available locally, but is also frequently contracted out.

This suggested approach can be modified based on local priorities and comfort level of the transplant team – for example, in an area with high prevalence of hemoglobinopathies and/or aplastic anemia, an initial focus on allogeneic rather than autologous transplantation may be advisable, especially if key personnel have prior experience in managing allogeneic HCT recipients. Although this chapter will not go into the details of setting up a cellular therapy program, the infrastructure and personnel established for a HCT program can also serve the needs of cellular therapy recipients. Overall, there is significant overlap in resources needed for autologous and allogeneic transplantation and cellular therapies.

Various models of care delivery can be pursued as an HCT program is being developed, and they can evolve as the program grows [16]. In this context, it is also important to understand the flow of a patient who is referred for and comes through the transplantation process (Fig. 13.1). When a program is in early stages of inception and volumes are rather small, the team and resources focused towards HCT can be shared by other cancer services. However, as the program matures and volumes increase, there may be a need to have personnel and resources dedicated towards hematologic malignancies and HCT, and ultimately in the setting of a high-volume program, HCT only.

In a report from the WBMT [7], the following elements were identified as highest priority and thus essential elements for development of an HCT program:

- Institution (or hospital leadership) support to develop a transplant program.
- Leadership by a hematologist, oncologist, or immunologist as a medical director.
- Nursing staff trained in handling chemotherapy and infection control.
- Availability of irradiated blood and platelets.

Referral	Pre-Transplant	Early Post-Transplant*	Late Post-Transplant*
- Evaluation of indication and candidacy for HCT - Evaluation for need for additional therapy - Evaluation for appropriate timing of HCT - Recipient HLA typing (allogeneic HCT) - Donor search and HLA typing (allogeneic HCT)	- HCT workup - Patient education - Caregiver assessment and education - Psychosocial assessment - Arrangement of additional resources (e.g., local lodging, transportation) - Assessment of donor suitability (allogeneic HCT) - Mobilization and collection of HPCs (autologous HCT) - Donor hematopoietic progenitor cell collection (allogeneic HCT)	- Conditioning regimen administration - HPC infusion - Inpatient or outpatient monitoring through engraftment - Outpatient monitoring for recovery and complications post-engraftment - Monitoring for acute graft-versus-host disease - Disease surveillance	- Outpatient monitoring for recovery and late complications - Monitoring for chronic graft-versus-host disease - Surveillance, screening, and management of late complications - Disease surveillance and maintenance therapy - Management of disease relapse - Care coordination with local clinicians

*Early post-transplant phase typically begins at initiation of conditioning regimen and lasts through 100 days post-transplantation and subsequently transitions to the late post-transplant phase

Fig. 13.1 Typical flow of HCT recipient (HPC denotes hematopoietic progenitor cells)

- Laboratory services with blood cell counter, chemistry, microbiology testing for bacteria and fungus, pre-transplant infectious disease markers.
- Access to standard radiology and computed tomography.
- Availability of chemotherapy, antiemetics, and broad-spectrum antibiotics.
- Availability of interventional radiology expertise for insertion of indwelling central venous catheters.
- Access to HLA typing laboratory (for allogeneic HCT).
- Monitoring levels of calcineurin inhibitors (for allogeneic HCT).
- Availability of antivirals and antifungal for treatment (for allogeneic HCT).
- Prophylaxis and agents to prevent and treat graft-versus-host disease (GVHD, for allogeneic HCT).

The WBMT report also outlines preferred and ideal elements for developing an HCT program. With this foundation, HCT programs can evolve as they gain experience and grow and can add on personnel and infrastructure as they care for increasingly complex patients and perform more sophisticated transplantation procedures. Other guidelines are also available that can be used as a platform to define the required elements as a new HCT program is considered [17].

HCT Program Infrastructure

A good starting point for considering infrastructure and personnel requirements for an HCT program are FACT/JACIE standards. Table 13.1 describes the minimum infrastructure requirements for setting up an HCT program. It is not necessary for all of these resources to be available within the institution that offers HCT, since some of these services can be contracted out (e.g., HLA typing, cell processing, apheresis, blood bank).

Table 13.1 Infrastructure requirements suggested for establishing an HCT program (examples below highlight requirements above what a typical resource may be structured for in a high-functional medical institution)

Service	Examples of infrastructure requirements
Outpatient clinic	Single patient examination rooms Infusion chairs
Inpatient unit	Private (single bed) rooms with isolation capability
Pharmacy	Pharmacy equipped to handle chemotherapeutic agents
	Access to specialized medications (e.g., immunosuppressants, antimicrobials)
Radiology	CT scan and MRI Interventional radiology services (e.g., placement of central venous catheters, biopsy)
Radiation oncology	Setup and experience in providing total body irradiation (if radiation-based conditioning regimens are planned)
Blood bank	Adequate red blood cell and platelet blood product support Ability to irradiate and leukocyte reduced blood products Ability to store/cryopreserve hematopoietic progenitor cell product Apheresis
Laboratory medicine	HLA lab Ability to perform HCT-specific tests (e.g., drug levels)
Microbiology	Ability to perform infectious disease markers Monitoring for CMV (antigen or PCR) Monitoring for other organisms (e.g., fungi, viruses)
Pathology	Expertise in hematopathology Flow cytometry Cytogenetics and molecular pathology
Emergency medicine	Emergency department with experience in handling cancer patients
Other services	Intensive care unit, including ventilator support Nephrology services, including dialysis Gastroenterology services, including endoscopy services Operating room services if bone marrow harvests are planned

In general, an HCT program is best served by a dedicated outpatient and inpatient area. FACT/JACIE standards for clinical programs require presence of designated areas that have adequate space and design that minimizes microbial contamination, and allows for patient isolation and administration of intravenous fluids, blood products, and medications. This approach has the benefit of consolidating personnel and enhancing their experience. Furthermore, there are some infrastructural advantages to this approach. For example, HCT units will frequently have laminar flow rooms or rooms with high-efficiency particle air (HEPA) filtration systems, which are most economically installed in a concentrated area. Depending on the existing layout for an institution, there may be value to having dedicated areas for procedures within the outpatient area (e.g., for bone marrow biopsy). Quality assurance is a major component of a high-functioning HCT program, and a specific area for caring for transplant recipients helps ensure that processes and outcomes are monitored appropriately.

Other hospital services are also critical for optimal care of HCT recipients. For example, specialized imaging services such as interventional radiology are necessary for placement of central venous catheters and organ biopsies (e.g., for GVHD), gastroenterology and endoscopy services for evaluation and diagnosis of GVHD and alimentary tract infections, intensive care services for management of patients who have hemodynamic compromise or need ventilator support, and nephrology services for dialysis. The pharmacy services should be able to handle and dispense high-dose chemotherapy medications. Similarly, in addition to providing routine support for cancer patients, laboratory, pathology, microbiology, and transfusion medicine services need to evolve to support HCT recipients. For example, patients who are going through the transplantation process need monitoring for levels of calcineurin inhibitors and monitoring for CMV. If the center is planning to pursue allogeneic transplantation, the laboratory needs to be equipped to test (or send out to another lab) HLA typing and donor-specific antibodies and conduct chimerism testing post-transplantation. The blood bank should have a process for ensuring adequate blood product support for the HCT program, including ability to irradiate and leucocyte reduce blood products. Blood banks will often provide apheresis and hematopoietic progenitor cell (HPC) storage/cryopreservation services for HCT programs. Obtaining and maintaining accreditation from national organizations (e.g., American Association of Blood Banks (AABB), American Society for Histocompatibility and Immunogenetics (ASHI), European Federation for Immunogenetics (EFI), College of American Pathologists (CAP)) ensures that ancillary services have the required infrastructure, processes, and experience to support the HCT program.

HCT Program Personnel

Similar to infrastructure requirements, FACT/JACIE standards can lay the foundation for determining personnel required for an HCT program (Table 13.2). Ultimately, a high-functioning, experienced, and cohesive team is required to provide high-quality and interdisciplinary care to HCT recipients. Additional training and qualifications specifically in HCT are often preferred for many personnel who participate in the care of transplant patients.

FACT/JACIE standards require an HCT program to have a dedicated clinical program director with background training in hematology, medical oncology, or immunology with at least 2 years of experience in direct clinical management of transplant patients. This individual is responsible for clinical and administrative operations and oversees care provided by the whole program. In addition, at least one other attending physician is recommended with one or more years of experience in the management of HCT recipients. It is not uncommon for programs to have physician trainees participate in the care of transplant patients. Many programs, especially in the United States, use advanced practice providers (APPs) such as nurse practitioners and physician assistants to provide care for their patients.

Table 13.2 Personnel requirements suggested for establishing an HCT program

Physician and related staff
   Clinical program director
   Additional attending physician
   Advanced practice provider
   Trainee physician
   Consulting specialists
   Palliative medicine specialists

Outpatient personnel
   Nurse/care coordinator
   Educator
   Financial navigator
   Social worker or psychosocial clinician
   Pharmacist
   Physical therapists or physiotherapist

Inpatient personnel
   Nurse
   Social worker
   Pharmacist
   Physical therapists or physiotherapist

Other personnel
   Program manager or administrator
   Data coordinator
   Quality manager
   Dietician
   Research nurses and coordinators

Nursing staff with experience in management of HCT patients are a critical component of a successful HCT program. In the outpatient setting, nurses may be involved in patient and donor education, pretransplant testing, and posttransplant care coordination. On the inpatient side, they need to be experienced in the administration of high-dose preparative regimens, infusion of HPC and blood products, providing supportive care, and management of various transplant related complications.

Several other team members are critical for safe and optimal care of HCT recipients. Some examples of such personnel include pharmacists and social workers. Pharmacists with experience in transplantation and dedicated to HCT program are in fact required per FACT/JACIE standards. There is guidance available from the American Society for Transplantation and Cellular Therapy (ASTCT) on the role of pharmacists in an HCT program, which can serve as a foundation for defining their role in patient care, education, research, and quality improvement [18, 19]. Social workers or psychosocial clinicians can assist in pretransplant evaluation of donors and recipients, facilitate with lodging, transportation, financial grants, and other social needs of patients, and screen and triage psychological complications. Guidance that defines the role of social workers in facilitating and optimizing the care of HCT recipients has been published [20].

In addition to clinical staff, several other personnel play a key role in the functioning of an HCT program. FACT/JACIE standards require a clinical program quality manager whose role involves establishing standard operating procedures and maintaining systems and processes to ensure they are followed and the program is in compliance. These individuals often manage data operations, especially for smaller programs. Additional personnel for data management and research may be required, depending on whether there is the availability and interest in pursuing research. It is advantageous for centers to submit data to a central registry such as the Center for International Blood and Marrow Transplant Research (CIBMTR) or the European Society for Blood and Marrow Transplantation (EBMT) (see below), and additional personnel for data capture and reporting may be needed for this purpose.

Several physician specialists and other clinicians outside the HCT team are also required for the care of HCT recipients. Some examples of these specialties include surgery, pulmonary medicine, intensive care, gastroenterology, nephrology, infectious diseases, cardiology, pathology, psychiatry, radiology, radiation oncology, ophthalmology, dentistry, dermatology, and palliative care.

The expertise of personnel may change and evolve as the HCT program grows. For example, the skillset for managing allogeneic HCT recipients may be different than autologous HCT recipients, since expertise in managing issues such as fungal and viral infections and GVHD is required. Similarly, the models of care and roles for specific personnel may change with the growth of the program – for instance, an outpatient nurse position may get further specialized as the number of patients transplanted increases, with separate nurses focusing on donor search and pretransplant evaluation, patient education, and post-transplant care coordination. An institution has to recognize that there is no one standard model of care for a transplant program, and the roles, types, and number of personnel depends on local infrastructure, priorities, and existing resources.

Quality Management

A successful HCT program requires a robust quality management program to monitor its performance, ascertain consistency of established processes, identify areas for improvement, implement corrective action for deficiencies, establish a culture of continuous improvement, and demonstrate operational effectiveness to internal and external entities. Recognizing its importance, FACT/JACIE standards require that HCT programs identify an individual who serves as quality manager and that programs have a quality management plan. Given its complexity, use of healthy donors, and economic impact, transplantation tends to be highly regulated by many countries, and the quality program also supports compliance with requirements laid out by national regulatory authorities.

A successful quality program requires collaborative and interdisciplinary interactions between all stakeholders who are involved in the care of HCT recipients (Fig. 13.2). The program director and the quality manager ultimately maintain responsibility for engaging these stakeholder groups and ensure cohesive interactions that focus on continuous program improvement and high-quality patient care.

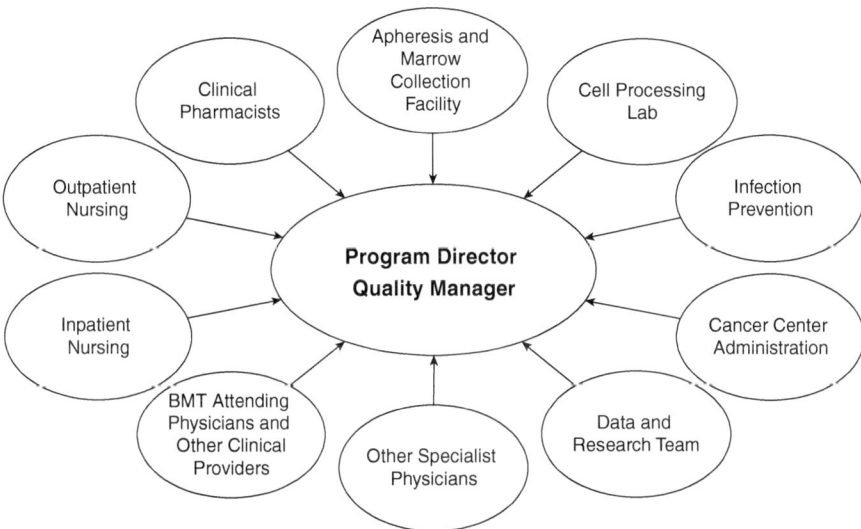

Fig. 13.2 Example of various stakeholders required for an interdisciplinary and effective quality program

The FACT/JACIE standards are a good starting point to define the scope of the quality program. How the quality program is structured and what aspects of transplant recipient care are under its oversight can vary by program. The HCT program should also establish certain benchmarks where it can meaningfully review its performance and use those data as the foundation for program review and improvement (Table 13.3). In general, examples of some areas that may be under the purview of a quality program include:

- Personnel onboarding, continuing education, and maintaining competency – the quality manager can ensure that HCT program personnel are assigned relevant educational modules and complete all requirements for maintaining educational and professional competency as it relates to transplantation.
- Facility compliance – to meet accreditation and other regulatory standards, facility and equipment routinely used for the care of HCT recipients often needs continuous monitoring (e.g., functioning and maintenance of apheresis machine and cryogenic storage).
- Documentation – HCT programs are required to maintain standard operating procedures (SOPs) that describe their processes and clinical guidelines, and the quality manager's responsibilities typically include their development and maintenance, and ensuring that the HCT program and its personnel are in compliance.
- Audits – One aspect of quality assurance is to review compliance with various HCT program data, processes and SOPs, and the quality manager typically conducts these audits with help from other program personnel.
- Adverse event monitoring – The complexity of HCT procedure and processes does increase risk of adverse events, and one role of the quality manager is to

Table 13.3 Sample metrics to monitor as part of HCT Program quality plan

Clinical program outcome metrics
    Overall survival (100 days, 1 year)
    Non-relapse mortality (100 days, 1 year)
    Acute GVHD rate (100 days)
    Chronic GVHD rate (1 year)
    Length of stay for transplant hospitalization
    Readmission rate
    Engraftment and graft failure rates

Patient safety metrics
    Rate of center line-associated blood stream infection
    Rate of *C. difficile* infections
    Rate of chemotherapy safety error events
    Rate of other medication safety error events
    Rate of falls
    Rate of compliance with hand hygiene
    Rate of mislabeled specimen events
    Rate of infusion reactions

Apheresis collection facility metrics
    Days required for adequate PBSC collection
    Rate of positive culture for HPC product
    CD34 collection efficiency
    Rate of central line use (in healthy donors)
    Rate of exceptional releases from apheresis
    Rate of serious adverse events

establish processes for monitoring and reporting of expected and unexpected adverse events along with their remediation.
- Continuous improvement – Another aspect of the quality program is to provide tools and data for improving processes and outcomes, and the quality manager can lead these efforts under guidance form the HCT program director.

The quality aspects for the HCT program along with the resources needed to manage them will typically evolve with program growth, with implementation of high-risk allogeneic transplant programs necessitating more complex quality-related processes and procedures. Newer cellular therapy modalities add to the complexity, as exemplified by FDA-approved CAR T products which have somewhat different requirements depending on the company providing the cells.

Data and Research

HCT and cellular therapy are highly innovative and rapidly evolving fields. An active HCT program can serve as a platform for academic development and knowledge generation. In addition, data captured for research can be repurposed and support the program from quality and clinical management standpoints.

To support these efforts, we do recommend one or more data managers be incorporated within the HCT program structure from the outset. For an early program still in its establishment phase, the individual overseeing quality can perform many of the duties expected of a data manager. However, as the program grows and becomes busier, investment into a data capture and management software solution along with personnel and resources to support them can be an excellent investment. Some HCT programs use simple systems to capture and manage data, whereas more sophisticated systems can also integrate into the clinical workflow for programs and possibly connect with the institutions' electronic medical record.

Data capture on patient demographics, disease status, transplant regimen, and posttransplant complications and outcomes can serve several purposes. Since HCT is a highly regulated field, these data can be used to provide aggregate information on transplant activity and outcomes to regulatory and accreditation organizations. Payers and policy makers may also request access to these aggregate data to evaluate HCT program capabilities and performance. The data collected often support quality management aspects of the program. It is advantageous to report data to central registries such as the CIBMTR, the EBMT, or another national or international registry, since it provides a foundation for meaningful data that a center needs to capture, provides opportunities for HCT program faculty to participate in collaborative research and discovery, and can help benchmark HCT program data and outcomes with other similar programs. Along with collection of data, there needs to exist robust mechanisms to ensure that the data are accurate. Besides having well-trained and high-functioning data coordinators, regular audits can help in ascertaining the quality of data collected.

Cellular Therapy

Recently, there has been significant interest in the application of non-HCT cellular therapies such as CAR T-cell therapy. Several products are now approved and commercially available for the treatment of lymphoma (axicabtagene ciloleucel, brexucabtagene autoleucel, and tisagenlecleucel), acute lymphoblastic leukemia (tisagenlecleucel), and myeloma (idecabtagene vicleucel). Several CAR T-cell and other cellular therapy products are under clinical investigation for the treatment of a spectrum of hematologic malignancies and solid tumors, and for nonmalignant indications. In essence, the clinical management, infrastructural, resource, personnel, process, and quality components are very similar to HCT, and transplant programs are a natural fit for administering standard of care and investigational cellular therapy products. FACT/JACIE standards are available for immune effector cell therapy and can serve as the foundation for setting up a cellular therapy program. An experienced transplant program should generally be able to offer these therapies within its existing infrastructure. As we look ahead, there will be an increasing use of cellular therapy for cancer and noncancer indications, and availability of these services within a cancer center will be necessary for provision on comprehensive cancer care services.

In conclusion, a successful HCT and cellular therapy program is a service line that indicates that a cancer center has the infrastructure and commitment to provide comprehensive cancer care services. It provides the opportunity to provide the complete spectrum of care for patients with advanced hematologic malignancies and other diseases. A successful program requires leadership and presence of a high-functioning clinical team in order to optimize patient experience and outcomes.

References

1. Gratwohl A, Pasquini MC, Aljurf M, et al. One million haemopoietic stem-cell transplants: a retrospective observational study. Lancet Haematol. 2015;2(3):e91–100.
2. Majhail NS, Chitphakdithai P, Logan B, et al. Significant improvement in survival after unrelated donor hematopoietic cell transplantation in the recent era. Biol Blood Marrow Transplant. 2015;21(1):142–50.
3. Majhail NS, Tao L, Bredeson C, et al. Prevalence of hematopoietic cell transplant survivors in the United States. Biol Blood Marrow Transplant. 2013;19(10):1498–501.
4. Hahn T, McCarthy PL Jr, Hassebroek A, et al. Significant improvement in survival after allogeneic hematopoietic cell transplantation during a period of significantly increased use, older recipient age, and use of unrelated donors. J Clin Oncol. 2013;31(19):2437–49.
5. McCarthy PL Jr, Hahn T, Hassebroek A, et al. Trends in use of and survival after autologous hematopoietic cell transplantation in North America, 1995-2005: significant improvement in survival for lymphoma and myeloma during a period of increasing recipient age. Biol Blood Marrow Transplant. 2013;19(7):1116–23.
6. Aljurf M, Weisdorf D, Hashmi SK, et al. Worldwide Network for Blood and Marrow Transplantation (WBMT) recommendations for establishing a hematopoietic stem cell transplantation program in countries with limited resources (Part II): clinical, technical and socioeconomic considerations. Hematol Oncol Stem Cell Ther. 2020;13(1):7–16.
7. Pasquini MC, Srivastava A, Ahmed SO, et al. Worldwide Network for Blood and Marrow Transplantation (WBMT) recommendations for establishing a hematopoietic cell transplantation program (Part I): minimum requirements and beyond. Hematol Oncol Stem Cell Ther. 2020;13(3):131–42.
8. Kanate AS, Majhail NS, Savani BN, et al. Indications for hematopoietic cell transplantation and immune effector cell therapy: guidelines from the American Society for Transplantation and Cellular Therapy. Biol Blood Marrow Transplant. 2020;26(7):1247–56.
9. Duarte RF, Labopin M, Bader P, et al. Indications for haematopoietic stem cell transplantation for haematological diseases, solid tumours and immune disorders: current practice in Europe, 2019. Bone Marrow Transplant. 2019;54(10):1525–52.
10. Majhail NS, Jagasia M. Referral to transplant center for hematopoietic cell transplantation. Hematol Oncol Clin North Am. 2014;28(6):1201–13.
11. Besse KL, Preussler JM, Murphy EA, et al. Estimating demand and unmet need for allogeneic hematopoietic cell transplantation in the United States using geographic information systems. J Oncol Pract. 2015;11(2):e120–30.
12. Shah GL, Majhail N, Khera N, Giralt S. Value-based care in hematopoietic cell transplantation and cellular therapy: challenges and opportunities. Curr Hematol Malig Rep. 2018;13(2):125–34.

13. Snowden JA, McGrath E, Duarte RF, et al. JACIE accreditation for blood and marrow transplantation: past, present and future directions of an international model for healthcare quality improvement. Bone Marrow Transplant. 2017;52(10):1367–71.
14. Majhail NS, Mau LW, Chitphakdithai P, et al. Transplant center characteristics and survival after allogeneic hematopoietic cell transplantation in adults. Bone Marrow Transplant. 2020;55(5):906–17.
15. Snowden JA, Saccardi R, Orchard K, et al. Benchmarking of survival outcomes following haematopoietic stem cell transplantation: a review of existing processes and the introduction of an international system from the European Society for Blood and Marrow Transplantation (EBMT) and the Joint Accreditation Committee of ISCT and EBMT (JACIE). Bone Marrow Transplant. 2020;55(4):681–94.
16. Majhail NS, Mau LW, Chitphakdithai P, et al. National survey of hematopoietic cell transplantation center personnel, infrastructure, and models of care delivery. Biol Blood Marrow Transplant. 2015;21(7):1308–14.
17. Faulkner L, Verna M, Rovelli A, et al. Setting up and sustaining blood and marrow transplant services for children in middle-income economies: an experience-driven position paper on behalf of the EBMT PDWP. Bone Marrow Transplant. 2021;56(3):536–43.
18. Clemmons AB, Alexander M, DeGregory K, Kennedy L. The hematopoietic cell transplant pharmacist: roles, responsibilities, and recommendations from the ASBMT Pharmacy Special Interest Group. Biol Blood Marrow Transplant. 2018;24(5):914–22.
19. Clemmons A. The hematopoietic cell transplant pharmacist: a call to action. Pharmacy (Basel). 2020;8(1):3.
20. Stickney Ferguson S, Randall J, Dabney J, et al. Perceived workforce challenges among clinical social workers in hematopoietic cell transplantation programs. Biol Blood Marrow Transplant. 2018;24(5):1063–8.

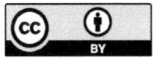

Chapter 14
Building Quality from the Ground Up in a Cancer Center

Arslan Babar and Alberto J. Montero

Background

In a landmark article in 1966 [1], Avedis Donabedian, one of the pioneers of quality improvement in medicine, proposed a structural framework for assessing quality in healthcare. According to this framework, quality in healthcare is evaluated on three different dimensions: structure, process, and outcome. This framework remains relevant today and is still an extremely useful model for assessing quality in medicine.

Structure, in Donabedian's model, is the context of where and how care is delivered and paid for. This includes facilities, equipment, people who provide the care, and the ways care is paid for. Process involves the interactions between patients and providers along the entire continuum of care—in other words, the processes by which providers and hospital systems can ensure the safety and well-being of patients. Outcome, the third dimension, is what most think about when they consider quality in health care—that is, the end result or effect of the care on the health status of individuals and entire populations. Example would be unplanned hospital readmissions, or five-year survival rates in patients with breast cancer.

In later work, Donabedian expanded his quality framework into the "seven pillars of quality": efficacy, effectiveness, efficiency, optimality, acceptability, legitimacy, and equity [2, 3]. The three components and seven pillars have served as the backbone of quality improvement in subsequent decades. A useful summary of

A. Babar
Taussig Cancer Institute, Cleveland Clinic Foundation, Cleveland, OH, USA
e-mail: Babara@ccf.org

A. J. Montero (✉)
Breast Cancer Program, UH Seidman Cancer Center, Diana Hyland Chair for Breast Cancer, Cleveland, OH, USA

CWRU School of Medicine, Cleveland, OH, USA
e-mail: Alberto.Montero@uhhospitals.org

© The Author(s) 2022
M. Aljurf et al. (eds.), *The Comprehensive Cancer Center*,
https://doi.org/10.1007/978-3-030-82052-7_14

Donabedian's work was published in *NEJM* in 2016, on the fiftieth anniversary of his seminal article [4].

Reports from the Institute of Medicine (IOM) in the United States in 1990, 1999, and 2001 adopted Donabedian's framework in their analyses and their recommendations for implementation. The first of these reports, *Medicare: A Strategy for Quality Assurance* [5], called for the creation of a Medicare Program to Assure Quality (MPAQ) and largely employed Donabedian's structure-process-outcome framework. The second report, *Ensuring Quality Cancer Care* [6], applied improvement principles specifically to cancer care, creating a twenty-first century framework for quality measurement in oncology, building on Donabedian's original triad of structure, process, and outcome. The 2001 report, *Crossing the Quality Chasm* [7], meanwhile, highlighted six core aims (similar to Donabedian's seven pillars) for quality in health care: safe, effective, patient-centered, timely, efficient, and equitable. Subsequent reports from IOM/NAM have continued to build on this work [8].

Quality improvement in cancer care is especially urgent today, given the rising global incidence of cancer and soaring drug costs. The annual cost of care for a cancer patient is four times that for a noncancer patient in the United States [9]. The cost of cancer care is rising, and one major study has predicted a U.S. cancer survivorship expenditure growth rate of 1.99% over the period from 2015 to 2030 ($183 billion to $246 billion, inclusive of care and drug costs) [10]. Globally, the burden of cancer is expected to rise. The World Health Organization's (WHO) International Agency for Research on Cancer predicts a global increase in new cancer cases from 18.1 to 29.5 million from 2018 to 2040 (2.25% yearly growth rate), if rates remain constant, due only to population growth and demographic trends [11]. The increase is heterogeneous with respect to location and cancer type. For example, from 2013 to 2035, colorectal cancer cases are expected to increase in Australia by 59% and in the United States by 28%, while the number of deaths globally is expected to increase by 60% for colon cancer and 71% for rectal cancer [12].

The updated IOM report recognized the challenges faced by cancer care delivery. According to the IOM report, the number of adults older than 65 is rapidly increasing. Because the majority of cancer diagnoses and deaths occur in this demographic, the incidence of cancer is expected to increase 45% by 2030. Taken together, the rapid increase in the geriatric population, steady increase in the incidence of age-related cancers, and rapidly evolving treatment landscape underscore the importance of multidisciplinary cancer care. Consequently, a cancer center model appears to be the best model for ensuring high-quality cancer care in a patient-centered manner.

High-quality cancer care is characterized by the following features [13]:

- Prioritizes the safety of patients, through creation of processes that minimize harm and medical errors.
- Creates a culture that promotes evidence-based care and continuous improvement of current practices.
- Maintains a patient-centered focus, and factor in personal and cultural needs.

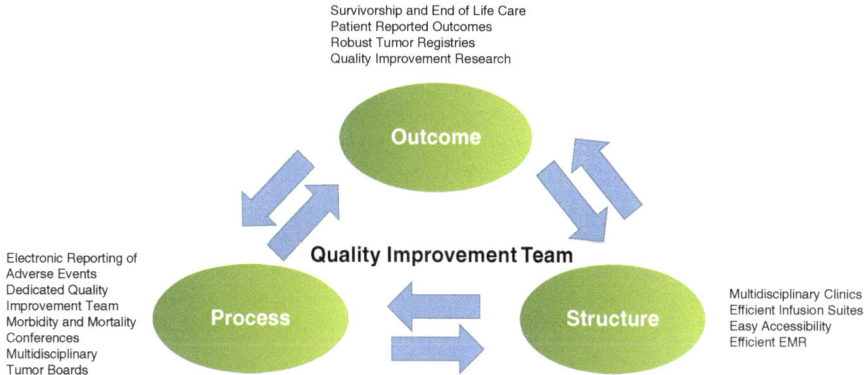

Fig. 14.1 Proposed quality of care model for cancer centers

- Practices time efficiency, and minimize any delays that would be harmful to the patient and/or the caregivers.
- Avoids any form of waste, including supplies, equipment, ideas, and human resources.
- Ensures fairness and equity among all patients without discrimination.

Toward this end, when thinking about how to build a high-quality cancer center, Donabedian's model is particularly useful in considering these essential components (Fig. 14.1).

Structure

In Donabedian's model, structure refers to the context of where the care is delivered. Cancer care is complex and multidisciplinary. Therefore, a structural feature of quality cancer care is to have all the necessary personnel and physical resources in close proximity. This proximity permits cancer patients to see multiple specialists on the same day, thereby reducing the time to treatment. Moreover, having multiple resources, such as radiation and infusion suites, in proximity permits patients to receive care without needing to travel long distances to a new facility. Proximity of providers also facilitates communication between specialists and helps to break down barriers between different departments (e.g., surgery and medical oncology) that serve as impediments to quality in medicine.

For these reasons, multidisciplinary clinics (MDC) are a hallmark of quality and patient-centered cancer care. Multidisciplinary clinics have been shown to reduce time to treatment, decrease number of visits, improve communication between teams, increase patient satisfaction, improve quality of life, and even improve survival [14].

Patients, families, and caregivers are at the heart of high-quality cancer care. High-quality cancer care should, therefore, ensure that the needs of the patients and their caregivers are met, which should include support in making informed decisions that are based on evidence-based medicine and, more importantly, align with patients' values and expectations. Cancer centers must assist their patients and families to comprehend the overall prognosis, benefits of treatments, and possible harms fully; provide palliative care, social support, and psychological support; and estimate cancer treatment costs accurately. In the setting of terminal cancer, resources that emphasize the importance of end-of-life care to maximize quality of life should be readily available.

Additionally, a structural hallmark of a high-quality cancer center are the professionals who provide care to patients. These include surgical, medical, and radiation oncologists, pathologists, palliative care physicians, oncology nurses, psychosocial workers, pharmacists, and other specialties that are routinely involved in providing cancer care. All providers should work together and effectively communicate, ensuring seamless transitions for patients and their families. All healthcare workers should also possess appropriate proficiencies and make appropriate treatment recommendations based on patients' and families' wishes. Roles should be clearly defined, and responsibilities assigned, with clear expectations from each member. There should be mutual trust between members, and communication should be effective. A cancer center should help continually improve communication skills among the staff with patients.

Health information technology systems also play an integral role in ensuring a high-quality cancer center. The electronic medical record (EMR) should be efficient and able to provide information to patients and healthcare providers in an effective manner, and it ideally should be structured to promote continuous improvement.

Finally, a cancer center needs a team of quality professionals—including a physician lead, a nursing lead, and a nonphysician with a quality improvement background—who structurally comprise the core team that is tasked to help drive quality throughout the entire cancer center.

Process

Medical errors are common in medicine. A medical error is a preventable adverse effect of medical care, whether or not it is evident or harmful to the patient [15]. A 2013 study estimated that medical errors were the third leading cause of death in the United States, after heart disease and cancer, accounted for approximately 210,000 and 440,000 deaths annually [16]. The nine most common medical errors in the United States in 2014, in order of frequency, were adverse drug events, catheter-associated urinary tract infection (CAUTI), central line–associated bloodstream infection (CLABSI), injury from falls and immobility, obstetrical adverse events, pressure ulcers, surgical site infections (SSI), venous thrombosis (blood clots), and ventilator-associated pneumonia (VAP) [17].

The high complexity of cancer care and the morbidity of many cancer treatments greatly increase the potential for medical error, unfavorable outcomes, and system failure. Therefore, it is imperative for cancer centers to create a culture of safety, where all providers are expected to report and disclose errors due to the complexity of narrow therapeutic index of many cancer treatments. To support a culture of reporting medical errors, cancer centers should have an electronic reporting system in place that facilitates the reporting of adverse events by all members of the healthcare team. There should be a dedicated team comprised of physicians, nurses, and administrative staff who deal with adverse event reporting and are trained in performing root cause analyses. This electronic platform should help to identify trends over time, enabling quality improvement work.

Morbidity and mortality (M&M) conferences are another vital tool that cancer centers should routinely use to improve overall quality of care [18]. These conferences provide a venue where errors and adverse events from individual cases can be discussed and process issues identified.

In addition to M&M conferences, multidisciplinary tumor boards (MDTB) are an integral part of cancer care management, where experts from various domains of oncology discuss and present newly diagnosed patients. Research has shown that MDTBs lead to more accurate diagnosis, more accurate staging, and more appropriate treatments [19].

To ensure high-quality care, cancer centers must create a system of continuous improvement where key quality metrics are measured along the entire continuum of cancer care. An organization cannot consistently deliver quality products or services without creating a system that promotes continuous improvement as well as self-improvement of employees. An organization cannot mandate excellence simply by slogans and unrealistic decrees by management [20].

Therefore, in order to hardwire quality and excellence, cancer center leadership must create an environment where processes are continuously improved, and those closest to the work are empowered to make changes that will lead to care of the highest possible quality for all patients. Continuous improvement is impossible without identification and measurement of key quality metrics. It is essential that those closest to the work (nurses, physicians, pharmacists, etc.), who are the content experts, help with deciding what key metrics to focus on and how best to measure them. Leadership is responsible with providing the infrastructure to measure key metrics and provide resources to permit continuous improvement of all cancer center processes with the goal of improving the quality of care for all patients.

Fortunately, American Society of Clinical Oncology (ASCO), National Comprehensive Cancer Network (NCCN), and international oncology organizations have developed a wealth of quality metrics for cancer centers to use, helping to simplify the work of selecting and defining metrics (Table 14.2). For example, NCCN advances its mission to improve and facilitate quality, effective, efficient, and accessible cancer care through creation and continuous update of clinical practice guideline, thereby facilitating creation of a reliable source for patients, clinicians, payers, and other healthcare decision-makers. Table 14.1 presents quality measures selected by NCCN's Quality and Outcomes Committee (Table 14.2).

Table 14.1 Quality measures selected by the NCCN quality and outcomes committee [23]

Cancer	Quality metrics
Breast	Patients should receive breast/chest wall plus regional lymph node radiation if they have M0 disease or involvement of ≥4 axillary lymph nodes.
Breast	Patients who have been cured of breast cancer should not have tumor markers performed during the follow-up surveillance period.
Colorectal	Patients with rectal cancer should undergo staging CT chest, abdomen, pelvis and pelvic MRI with contrast or endorectal ultrasound before surgery.
Colorectal	Carcinoembryonic antigen should be performed every 6 months for 5 years for patients with resected pathological stage II and III colorectal cancer.
Lung	Patients with newly diagnosed metastatic non-small cell lung cancer should have a palliative medicine consult within 8 weeks of diagnosis.
Prostate	All patients in high-risk prostate cancer group who undergo radiation should be treated with androgen deprivation therapy.
Prostate	Patients who have undergone surgery or radiation for localized prostate cancer should be evaluated for sexual dysfunction and urinary incontinence.
Prostate	Patients with prostate cancer should have prostate specific antigen measured every 12 months to monitor recurrence of disease.
Cross-cancer	Cancer stage should be documented. Performance status should be documented before starting systemic therapy. Percentage of patients with cancer admitted to intensive care unit in the last 30 days of life. Patients who smoke should be offered smoking cessation counselling. Number of patients undergoing chemotherapy in the last 14 days of life. Number of patients dying from cancer in the acute care setting. Chemotherapy given within 30 days of end of life.

Outcome

In medicine, there is a much greater focus on outcomes than processes. This is understandable, since the overall goal of treating any cancer is ultimately cure. However, any outcome is the culmination of many processes, and improving an outcome is nearly impossible without a thorough understanding of all the processes involved that led to a specific outcome. Take, for example, the diagnosis and subsequent treatment of early stage breast cancer. This involves many processes, including breast cancer screening, radiographic interpretation, biopsy of suspicious lesions, pathologic interpretation, surgical management, selection of appropriate chemo- and endocrine therapy, radiation oncology, management of treatment-related toxicities, and cancer survivorship. Five-year breast cancer survival is a culmination of all of these processes, as well as others. To improve this outcome metric requires identification of key improvements in many or all of these processes.

This is not to say that outcome measures are not important. Indeed, they are extremely important. However, outcomes cannot be viewed as independent of processes, since they are completely dependent on them. Additionally, survival outcomes for a cancer center cannot be viewed in isolation of the populations that they serve. Population and socioeconomic factors can influence survival, independent of quality of medical care. For example, breast cancer mortality has been shown to correlate positively with socioeconomic factors that vary quite substantially across

Table 14.2 Selected resources on cancer care quality

Organization	Description	Link
American Academy of hospice and palliative medicine (AAHPM)	Resources and tools to address quality and patient safety in hospice and palliative care setting	http://aahpm.org/education/quality
American Society of Clinical Oncology (ASCO)	Information on ASCO quality programs, guidelines, chemotherapy safety standards, and quality oncology practice initiative (QOPI), and registry (CancerLinQ)	https://practice.asco.org/quality-improvement
American Society of Hematology (ASH)	Quality care resources specific to nonmalignant and malignant hematologic diseases	https://www.hematology.org/education/clinicians/guidelines-and-quality-care
American Society for Radiation Oncology (ASTRO)	List of quality measures specific to radiation oncology	https://www.astro.org/Daily-Practice/QPP/Measures/Inventory
Commission on Cancer (CoC)	Information on CoC standards to facilitate quality cancer care delivery	https://www.facs.org/quality-programs/cancer/coc
Foundation for the Accreditation of cellular therapy (FACT)	Quality standards for hematopoietic cell transplantation and cellular therapies	http://www.factwebsite.org/
American College of Surgeons (ACS)	National Accreditation Program for breast centers (NAPBC)	https://www.facs.org/Quality-Programs/NAPBC/Standards
National Comprehensive Cancer Network (NCCN)	List of high-priority and high-impact cancer quality measures proposed by NCCN	https://jnccn.org/view/journals/jnccn/18/3/article-p250.xml
National Quality Forum (NQF)	Cancer care quality measures endorsed by NQF	http://www.qualityforum.org/Cancer.aspx
Oncology Nursing Society (ONS)	ONS resources on quality cancer care	https://www.ons.org/make-difference/quality-improvement

countries and that are associated with economic development and social/lifestyle factors [21].

In order to measure long-term cancer outcomes, cancer centers need to have a robust tumor registry that can track outcomes among the cancer patients that they serve. These long-term outcomes would need to be stratified to factor in medical comorbidities and socioeconomic factors. Ideally, these data should be benchmarked to national data if available. This would require statistical and epidemiologic support that may not be readily available to all cancer centers but would be of great value, particularly when thinking about where the greatest opportunities are for improvement of cancer outcomes.

Patient satisfaction is also an important outcome that cancer centers must reliably track. Validated patient questionnaires that are provided to patients and their families are a key way to capture the voice of the patient and to identify areas of strength and areas where improvements must be made. Creating a culture of patient-centered care requires honest feedback from patients.

Another important outcome measure is patient-reported outcomes (PROs). Symptoms are common among patients receiving treatment for advanced cancers yet are undetected by clinicians up to half the time. There is growing interest in integrating electronic PROs into routine oncology practice for symptom monitoring. In a recent randomized trial, data integration of PROs into the routine care of patients with metastatic cancer was associated with a significant improvement in overall survival compared with usual care [22]. Earlier identification of emerging toxicities in patients enabled the oncology care team to intervene more rapidly before toxicities became more severe, enabling patients to stay on treatments longer and avoid unnecessary hospitalizations.

Conclusions

Quality in healthcare has three primary domains: structure, process, and outcome. This is the three-legged stool upon which clinical excellence sits. To successfully build quality from the ground up in a cancer center, first you need the right people. A quality team of professionals that is responsible for promoting a culture of excellence and quality improvement is needed. This small team should be comprised of physicians, nurses, pharmacists, data management, and quality improvement professionals. Responsibility should be delegated by executive leadership to this quality team to drive quality and foster a culture of quality improvement throughout the entire cancer center. High-quality care is synonymous with patient-centered care and is everyone's responsibility. Those who are closest to the patient and, therefore, have the greatest control over treatment decisions must be given the proper tools, education, and support to conduct quality improvement activities. Providers need access to timely data on relevant quality-related process and outcome measures, because improvement is practically impossible without formal longitudinal measurements. Fortunately, there are a wealth of validated oncology quality measures that have been created by ASCO, NCCN, and other organizations, which cancer centers can adapt.

References

1. Donabedian A. Evaluating the quality of medical care. Milbank Q. 2005;83(4):691–729. https://doi.org/10.1111/j.1468-0009.2005.00397.x.
2. Donabedian A. Explorations in quality assessment and monitoring. Health Administration Press; Ann Arbor, 1985.
3. Donabedian A. The seven pillars of quality. Arch Pathol Lab Med. 1990;114(11):1115–8.
4. Ayanian JZ, Markel H. Donabedian's lasting framework for health care quality. N Engl J Med. 2016;375(3):205–7. https://doi.org/10.1056/NEJMp1605101.
5. Institute of Medicine. Medicare: a strategy for quality assurance. National Academies Press; 1990. https://doi.org/10.17226/1547.
6. Institute of Medicine. Ensuring quality cancer care. National Academies Press; 1999. https://doi.org/10.17226/6467.
7. Institute of Medicine. Crossing the quality chasm: a new health system for the 21st century. National Academies Press; 2001. https://doi.org/10.17226/10027.

8. Institute of Medicine. Performance measurement: accelerating improvement. National Academies Press; 2006. https://doi.org/10.17226/11517.

9. Park J, Look KA. Health care expenditure burden of cancer care in the United States. Inq J Heal Care Organ Provision, Financ. 2019;56:004695801988069. https://doi.org/10.1177/0046958019880696.

10. Mariotto AB, Enewold L, Zhao J, Zeruto CA, Yabroff KR. Medical care costs associated with cancer survivorship in the United States. Cancer Epidemiol Biomark Prev. 2020;29(7):1304–12. https://doi.org/10.1158/1055-9965.EPI-19-1534.

11. Global Cancer Observatory. Cancer incidence in five continents time trends. Published 2020. Accessed July 4, 2020. https://ci5.iarc.fr/CI5plus/Pages/graph4_sel.aspx.

12. Araghi M, Soerjomataram I, Jenkins M, et al. Global trends in colorectal cancer mortality: projections to the year 2035. Int J Cancer. 2019;144(12):2992–3000. https://doi.org/10.1002/ijc.32055.

13. Levit L, Balogh E, Nass S, Ganz P, editors. Delivering high-quality cancer care: charting a new course for a system in crisis. Institute of Medicine; Washington (DC), 2013.

14. Horvath LE, Yordan E, Malhotra D, et al. Multidisciplinary care in the oncology setting: historical perspective and data from lung and gynecology multidisciplinary clinics. J Oncol Pract. 2010;6(6):e21–6. https://doi.org/10.1200/JOP.2010.000073.

15. Hofer TP, Kerr EA, Hayward RA. What is an error? Eff Clin Pract. 2000;3(6):261–9.

16. Makary MA, Daniel M. Medical error: the third leading cause of death in the US. BMJ. Published online May 2016:i2139. doi:https://doi.org/10.1136/bmj.i2139.

17. Carver N, Gupta V, Hipskind JE. Medical Error; 2020. In: StatPearls [Internet]. Treasure Island (FL): StatPearls Publishing; 2021. PMID: 28613514. Bookshelf ID: NBK430763.

18. Stover DG, Zerillo JA. Morbidity and mortality revisited: applying a new quality improvement paradigm in oncology. J Oncol Pract. 2015;11(3):e428–32. https://doi.org/10.1200/JOP.2014.003566.

19. Specchia ML, Frisicale EM, Carini E, et al. The impact of tumor board on cancer care: evidence from an umbrella review. BMC Health Serv Res. 2020;20(1):73. https://doi.org/10.1186/s12913-020-4930-3.

20. Gitlow H, Oppenhein A, Oppenheim R, Levine D. Quality management. 3rd ed. McGraw-Hill; New York, 2005.

21. Ji P, Gong Y, Jiang C, Hu X, Di G, Shao Z. Association between socioeconomic factors at diagnosis and survival in breast cancer: a population-based study. Cancer Med. 2020;9(5):1922–36. https://doi.org/10.1002/cam4.2842.

22. Basch E, Deal AM, Dueck AC, et al. Overall survival results of a trial assessing patient-reported outcomes for symptom monitoring during routine Cancer treatment. JAMA. 2017;318(2):197. https://doi.org/10.1001/jama.2017.7156.

23. D'Amico TA, Bandini LAM, Balch A, et al. Quality measurement in cancer care: a review and endorsement of high-impact measures and concepts. JNCCN J Natl Compr Cancer Netw. 2020;18(3):250–9. https://doi.org/10.6004/jnccn.2020.7536.

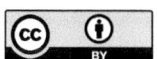

Chapter 15
Patient Resources in a Cancer Center

Farah Yassine and Mohamed A. Kharfan-Dabaja

Introduction

Treatment of cancer is complex and requires clinical expertise, close surveillance, and supportive therapies, among others, to help manage untoward side effects resulting from antineoplastic regimens. These therapies expose patients to adverse consequences such as increased organ toxicity that could adversely affect overall quality of life. For instance, childhood cancer survivors are at a higher risk of being unable to work or missing work because of poor health; they also report difficulties with obtaining insurance coverage, hence posing a challenge to adherence to optimal care [1]. A childhood cancer survivorship study showed that, in fact, survivors of childhood cancer spend a higher percentage of their income on medical expenses, adversely influencing their future health-seeking behavior and ultimately their treatment outcomes [2].

Novel targeted therapies with better toxicity profiles, vis-à-vis conventional chemotherapies, have become an integral part of treatment algorithms for various solid organ neoplasms and hematologic malignancies; they are already changing the treatment paradigm of various cancers [3–9]. However, these new therapies are expensive, especially when required to be taken for a long time [10, 11]. Unfortunately, patients with cancer are at high risk for substantial treatment-related costs owing to the high cost of these novel therapies. Apart from the high cost of therapies, availability of high-resolution genomic analysis of tumors, and other technologies, which are being used for more accurate diagnosis and prognostication have further added to the already elevated cost of treating cancer [12–14].

A recently published longitudinal study aimed at evaluating the impact of cancer on patient's debt in the United States found a substantial proportion incurring financial toxicity and asset depletion [15]. This is also the case for parents of children

F. Yassine · M. A. Kharfan-Dabaja (✉)

Division of Hematology-Oncology and Blood and Marrow Transplantation Program, Mayo Clinic, Jacksonville, FL, USA

e-mail: KharfanDabaja.Mohamed@mayo.edu

© The Author(s) 2022

M. Aljurf et al. (eds.), *The Comprehensive Cancer Center*,

https://doi.org/10.1007/978-3-030-82052-7_15

145

receiving anticancer therapies [1]. Below, we describe resources that are generally available to cancer patients to help cope with stressors associated with cancer care and to address their medical, financial, and spiritual needs, among others.

Available Resources

Education

Patient education is an essential requirement when developing a plan of cancer care. Education represents a continuum which is provided by several members of the treatment team, namely, hematologists/oncologists, advanced practice providers, nurses, nutritionists, and pharmacists, among others. Below, we describe available educational sources for patients, whether related to disease-specific, antineoplastic drugs and supportive therapy education.

Disease-Specific Education

Several cancer societies provide disease-specific education to patients with cancer. We summarize a small selected sample of societies and organizations:

(a) AA·MDS International Foundation (www.aamds.org).
(b) American Cancer Society (ACS) (www.cancer.org).
(c) International Myeloma Foundation (www.myeloma.org).
(d) Leukemia & Lymphoma Society (www.lls.org).
(e) Melanoma Research Foundation (www.melanoma.org).
(f) National Cancer Institute (NCI) (www.cancer.gov).
(g) Susan G. Komen, originally known as The Susan G. Komen Breast Cancer Foundation (ww5.komen.org).

Treatment Education

Below we summarize the most common types of antineoplastic therapies offered to patients apart from surgical tumor resection. We also highlight selected educational sources available to patients.

Conventional Chemotherapy

Conventional chemotherapy, alone or in combination with targeted therapies, remains an important treatment for various hematologic malignancies such as acute myeloid leukemia, acute lymphoblastic leukemia, lymphomas, breast, lung and colorectal cancer, among many others. Side effects associated with chemotherapy vary according to each agent, but generally result in bone marrow toxicity which manifests as pancytopenia and could increase risk of infections, and organ toxicity manifesting as alopecia, mucositis, enteritis, cardiomyopathy, hemorrhagic cystitis, and others. When severe toxicity ensues, it can result in death. Therefore, it is important to empower the patient with the necessary knowledge about commonly occurring side effects associated with specific chemotherapies to ensure more successful outcomes. This information is generally available in the package inserts that is found online for each specific antineoplastic agent. Others sources of information include the drug manufacturer, the ACS (www.cancer.org), and the NCI (www.cancer.gov).

Targeted Antineoplastic Therapies

Treatment of cancer has evolved over the past three decades. Nowadays, the backbone of anticancer treatments relies more heavily on targeted therapies, also known as precision medicine. It is a type of cancer treatment characterized by a more specific mode of action than conventional chemotherapy, through targeting specific genes and proteins involved in the growth and survival of cancer cells. It can either affect the tissue environment of cancer cells, or disrupt other key mechanisms essential for cancer growth and proliferation. Targeted therapies may be used as monotherapy; for example, in chronic lymphocytic leukemia and chronic myeloid leukemia; or in combination with other cancer treatments, namely, chemotherapy, surgery, or radiation in the case of solid tumors like lung, breast, and colorectal cancer. Below, we summarize several available online sources, apart from drug manufacturers, to educate patients about targeted therapies:

(a) The American College of Physicians (ACP) offers a library of patient education materials accessible through the following hyperlink: https://www.acponline.org/practice-resources/patient-and-interprofessional-education. ACP is currently replacing its online library with a new Patient and Interprofessional Partnership initiative, delivering high-quality, patient-centered, interprofessional education resources for internists, patients, and their clinical teams.

(b) UpToDate is another platform offering patient education through two levels of content: "The Basics," which are short overviews in easy-to-understand language aimed at answering important questions a patient may have about a medical topic; and "Beyond the Basics", which are extensive, more detailed reviews with some medical terminology. Information about targeted therapies is included within each type of cancer (https://www.uptodate.com/contents/table-of-contents/patient-education/cancer).

Following is a list of other selected resources for patient education on cancer-targeted therapies:

(a) The NCI: https://www.cancer.gov/about-cancer/treatment/types/targeted-therapies/targeted-therapies-fact-sheet

(b) My Cancer Genome: https://www.mycancergenome.org/content/page/overview-of-targeted-therapies-for-cancer/
(c) The ACS: https://www.cancer.org/treatment/treatments-and-side-effects/treatment-types/targeted-therapy.html
(d) The National Comprehensive Cancer Network (NCCN): https://www.nccn.org/patients/resources/life_with_cancer/treatment/targeted_therapy.aspx

Radiation Therapy

Since its discovery in the nineteenth century, radiation has been used in medicine through several applications [16]. In the field of cancer therapeutics, radiation therapy is one of the primary treatment modalities, exerting its action by directly killing cancer cells or causing DNA damage leading to tumor cell death [17]. Cancer patients also benefit from the option of radiation therapy in the palliative care setting, for example, to relieve pain caused by bone metastasis or cytoreducing large tumor masses obstructing the airway in head and neck cancers [18]. Constant advancements in this area enhanced the accuracy and quality of radiation delivery, increasing the survival rates for many patients [19]. Damage to healthy tissue near the treatment area results in multiple side effects, commonly skin problems (dryness, itching, blistering, or peeling), and fatigue [20]. Other side effects are site-specific: for instance, radiation therapy aimed at head and neck tumors causes dry mouth, difficulty swallowing, mouth sores, nausea, hair loss, and tooth decay [21]. Chest radiation may result in lung fibrosis, radiation pneumonitis, cough, fever, shortness of breath, and cardiovascular side effects [22]. Radiation therapy for solid malignancies is also associated with higher risk of acute leukemias and non-Hodgkin lymphomas [23].

Multiple educational resources for patients on radiation therapy benefits and side effects are available on the American Society for Radiation Oncology (ASTRO) website (https://www.astro.org/Patient-Care-and-Research/Patient-Education), including brief videos, patient brochures, and radiation therapy presentations. With the emergence of modern virtual environments, radiation therapy patient education has witnessed the rise of two recent educational tools, namely, the Virtual Environment for Radiotherapy Training (VERT) and the Patient Education And Radiotherapy Learning (PEARL). The VERT system relies on a three-dimensional interactive radiotherapy treatment room that replicates realistic movements, sounds and even a visible radiation beam, suitable for both patient education and residency training [24]. Similarly, the PEARL system uses common features including a virtual patient and treatment room environment, but with limited functionality as it is was solely conceived for the purpose of patient education [25]. Such rich visual displays and virtual environments constitute an innovative approach in radiation therapy patient education; however, they should be tuned to every cancer center's budget and capacity [26]. Their roles in supporting psychological and health-related patient outcomes are still under investigation.

Supportive Therapies

Availability of effective supportive therapies have facilitated timely administration of chemotherapy, chemoimmunotherapy, other targeted therapies, and radiation therapy. These supportive therapies include but are not limited to:

(a) Antiemetics to prevent nausea and vomiting.
(b) Antimicrobials (antibacterials, antifungals, and antivirals).
(c) Bisphosphonates or equivalents.
(d) Granulocyte-Colony stimulating factor (G-CSF) that stimulates the bone marrow to produce granulocytes.
(e) Intravenous fluids and electrolytes.
(f) Transfusion of blood products (red blood cell and platelets). In certain cases, patients may need infusions of fresh frozen plasma and cryoprecipitate.

Education about the side effects of these therapies are generally provided by treating hematologists/oncologists, nurses, and pharmacists. More detailed information is available at the manufacturer website or online drug package insert.

Supporting Services

Financial

Receiving a diagnosis of cancer not only imposes health-related challenges on the patient, but also results in "financial toxicity," a term coined to describe the financial hardships associated with the cost of cancer treatments. Patients experiencing financial burden elect to alter care to defray out-of-pocket expenses [27]. Moreover, high treatment expenditures have been associated with nonadherence and poor clinical outcomes in several studies [28–30] . Accordingly, the NCI recommends offering financial counselling services at cancer treatment centers to help patients and their families understand the scope of the problem and plan better on how to manage their anticipated expenses. In the absence of proper counselling, financial toxicity bears material and psychological consequences [31]. Material consequences are mainly monetary owing to reduction or loss of income, time away from work, depletion of savings, and ultimately bankruptcy [32]. Interestingly, cancer patients are twice more likely to file for bankruptcy as compared to people without cancer [33]. On the other hand, psychological consequences translate into increased stress, worry, and decreased quality of life [34]. As a result, cancer patients develop maladaptive coping behaviors to lower their cost of care, such as not showing up to scheduled visits, medication noncompliance, omitting doses, and neglecting refills [35].

Apart from financial counselling, patients are encouraged to seek financial help starting from oncology social workers, case managers, physicians, and oncology nurses who can provide referrals to financial resources and support services, in addition to contacts with national, regional, and local organizations for financial support. The ACS website also offers a list of programs and resources dedicated to help with cancer-related expenses like housing, transportation, caregiver expenses and food costs, accessible through the following hyperlink: https://www.cancer.org/ treatment/finding-and-paying-for-treatment/understanding-financial-and-legal-matters/managing-costs/programs-and-resources-to-help-with-cancer-related-expenses.html.

Palliative Care

Integration of palliative care into standard oncology management at the time of cancer diagnosis is essential for optimal quality care, based on evidence from clinical trials [36]. Palliative care services focus on approaching the patient as whole, communicating about goals of care while accounting for patient preferences [37]. This comprehensive approach addresses the quality of life, physical, psychological, emotional, religious, spiritual, and family concerns, as well as future care plans [38]. As such, offering palliative care to the patient and family caregivers confers additional emotional and psychological benefits by lowering levels of depression, caregiving burden, and psychological distress and anxiety [36].

Current professional guidelines recommend the integration of palliative care early in the disease course, and all throughout the treatment [39–41]. Palliative care is provided by specialists who work as part of a multidisciplinary care team that may include nurses, registered dieticians, pharmacists, chaplains, psychologists, and social workers, in conjunction with the oncology treatment team [38]. The American Society of Clinical Oncology (ASCO) offers a palliative care booklet (https://www.cancer.net/sites/cancer.net/files/palliative_care.pdf) to help cancer patients, their families, and caregivers understand options, find support, and ease the disease challenges. The NCI website also offers a wide platform to explain all about palliative care for patients and their families (https://www.cancer.gov/about-cancer/ advanced-cancer/care-choices/palliative-care-fact-sheet). Resources for program managers include the palliative care guide published by the World Health Organization that suggests steps for planning and implementing palliative care services at cancer treatment centers (https://apps.who.int/iris/bitstream/han dle/10665/250584/9789241565417-eng.pdf;jsessionid=45331C2A5976BE588817 9C10E4737A95?sequence=1).

While palliative care is provided at every step of treatment and at any stage of cancer, hospice care is a specific facet of palliative care only given to patients with advanced stages of cancer with a life expectancy of 6 months or less [42]. It shifts the focus from direct anticancer treatment to symptomatic relief. Consequently, the patient elects to stop chemotherapy, for example, and receive additional support in all other areas. Hospice is associated with less hospital-based end-of-life medical care, better quality of life, and improved caregiver outcomes [43–46], as well as better symptom relief and patient-goal attainment [47]. Therefore, encouraging earlier hospice enrollment may improve the end-of-life experiences for cancer patients and their families.

Social Workers

Social workers are essential members of the cancer care team. They help address a variety of issues which include, among others:

(a) Counseling for anxiety, depression, and other emotional aspects of cancer care.
(b) Identifying resources for financial assistance, compassionate drug assistance programs, disease support groups, or spiritual counseling, etc.
(c) Helping address and resolve transportation challenges.
(d) Education of caregivers about the disease.

Case Managers

A case manager is a healthcare professional who has vast clinical disease knowledge and a good understanding of the healthcare industry and payers' dynamics. A case manager is usually a nurse or nurse specialist who oversees all aspects of cancer care and helps patients navigate complex health insurance coverage issues, whether related to specific prescribed drug(s) or supportive services such as rehabilitation and skilled nursing facilities or nursing home placement, if indicated. Their ultimate goal is to optimize quality and cost-effective care in both hospital and outpatient cancer care settings.

Nutritional Therapists

Both the cancer and its treatment(s) contribute to cachexia. Cancer patients are at increased risk of malnutrition due to decreased food intake, adverse effects of cancer therapies, and increase in metabolic waste products. A wide range of negative sequelae result from malnutrition, including prolonged hospitalization, reduced response to cancer treatment, increased susceptibility to treatment toxicity, decreased activity, and impaired quality of life, culminating in a worse overall prognosis [48]. Therefore, proper diet plans and clinical nutrition are paramount. Nutritional therapists are registered dietitians that constitute another component of a cancer patient's care team. They work closely with patients and their families to develop realistic and appropriate diet plans during and after cancer treatment. It is widely agreed that early consultation with a nutritional therapist is beneficial for cancer patients [49, 50], even in advanced stages of the disease [51]. Nutritional support prevents malnutrition, thus improving treatment tolerance and prognosis, while maintaining the patient's functional activity and quality of life [52, 53]. As such, cancer centers provide consultation services with nutritional therapists and registered dieticians who help patients manage their nutritional concerns through personalized diet plans, safe food handling practices, weight management, multivitamin supplements, among others. Patients who fail to achieve adequate energy intake with oral nutritional supplements are offered enteral nutrition options, or tube feeding, provided they have normal gut function. In the absence of proper gut function or in case of patient refusal or intolerance due to nausea, vomiting or diarrhea, nutritional support is delivered through parenteral nutrition [52, 54–56].

Religious and Spiritual

In the context of patient-centered care, the holistic view of the patient should be addressed all along the cancer care continuum [57]. As such, support services must account for the patients religious and cultural beliefs, among others. Several tools have been developed to assess the religious and spiritual needs of cancer patients, among which are the Faith, Importance and Influence, Community, and Address (FICA) spiritual history tool [58, 59] and the Spiritual Needs Assessment for Patients (SNAP) questionnaire [60]. Once the specific needs are assessed, several interventions could be implemented. For instance, with the permission of the patient, a member of the patient's religious or spiritual community could be contacted [61]. The patient could be referred to hospital chaplaincy or psychosocial oncology providers, including oncology social workers, psychologists, or psychiatrists [61]. In other cases, members of the care team can intervene to address the religious and spiritual needs by offering narratives and psychotherapeutic interventions at bedside or during clinic visits [62]. Those interventions consist of a discussion of a short-term life review [63] and dignity talks [64] that enhance familial relationships with the patient and find purpose in the illness experience. Religious and spiritual support realizes particular prominence during end-of-life care, or once the patient resorts to hospice care.

Discussion

The field of cancer therapeutics has evolved dramatically over the past three decades bringing smarter therapies from the bench to the bedside. While novel therapies have revolutionized cancer care from the mechanistic standpoint, treatment remains complex requiring multiple players beyond hematologists/oncologists and nurses. Pharmacists, social workers, and case managers play an essential role in patient education about drugs and treatment complications, support needs, and financial aspects associated with care. The ultimate goal is to provide all needed support to help cancer patients with their fight against the disease.

Conflicts of Interests F.Y: No conflicts of interest to declare.

M.A.K-D: Discloses consultancy for Pharmacyclics and Daiichi Sankyo.

References

1. Nathan PC, et al. Financial hardship and the economic effect of childhood cancer survivorship. J Clin Oncol. 2018;36(21):2198–205.

2. Nipp RD, et al. Financial burden in survivors of childhood cancer: a report from the childhood cancer survivor study. J Clin Oncol. 2017;35(30):3474–81.
3. Paz-Ares L, et al. Pembrolizumab plus chemotherapy for squamous non-small-cell lung cancer. N Engl J Med. 2018;379(21):2040–51.
4. Nghiem PT, et al. PD-1 blockade with Pembrolizumab in advanced Merkel-cell carcinoma. N Engl J Med. 2016;374(26):2542–52.
5. Wolchok JD, et al. Overall survival with combined Nivolumab and Ipilimumab in advanced melanoma. N Engl J Med. 2017;377(14):1345–56.
6. Robert C, et al. Pembrolizumab versus Ipilimumab in advanced melanoma. N Engl J Med. 2015;372(26):2521–32.
7. Woyach JA, et al. Ibrutinib regimens versus Chemoimmunotherapy in older patients with untreated CLL. N Engl J Med. 2018;379(26):2517–28.
8. Zinzani PL, et al. Efficacy and safety of Pembrolizumab in relapsed/refractory primary mediastinal large B-cell lymphoma (rrPMBCL): updated analysis of the Keynote-170 phase 2 trial. Blood. 2017;130(Suppl 1):2833.
9. Wang ML, et al. Targeting BTK with ibrutinib in relapsed or refractory mantle-cell lymphoma. N Engl J Med. 2013;369(6):507–16.
10. Chen Q, et al. Economic burden of chronic lymphocytic leukemia in the era of oral targeted therapies in the United States. J Clin Oncol. 2017;35(2):166–74.
11. Shanafelt TD, et al. Impact of ibrutinib and idelalisib on the pharmaceutical cost of treating chronic lymphocytic leukemia at the individual and societal levels. J Oncol Pract. 2015;11(3):252–8.
12. Bejar R, et al. Clinical effect of point mutations in myelodysplastic syndromes. N Engl J Med. 2011;364(26):2496–506.
13. Yandell DW, et al. Oncogenic point mutations in the human retinoblastoma gene: their application to genetic counseling. N Engl J Med. 1989;321(25):1689–95.
14. Jamal-Hanjani M, et al. Tracking the evolution of non-small-cell lung cancer. N Engl J Med. 2017;376(22):2109–21.
15. Gilligan AM, et al. Death or debt? National Estimates of financial toxicity in persons with newly-diagnosed Cancer. Am J Med. 2018;131(10):1187–1199.e5.
16. Jean-Claude R, Nusslin F. Marie Curie's contribution to medical physics. Phys Med. 2013;29(5):423–5.
17. Abshire D, Lang MK. The evolution of radiation therapy in treating cancer. Semin Oncol Nurs. 2018;34(2):151–7.
18. Grewal AS, Jones J, Lin A. Palliative radiation therapy for head and neck cancers. Int J Radiat Oncol Biol Phys. 2019;105(2):254–66.
19. Chetty IJ, et al. Technology for Innovation in radiation oncology. Int J Radiat Oncol Biol Phys. 2015;93(3):485–92.
20. Yee C, et al. Radiation-induced skin toxicity in breast cancer patients: a systematic review of randomized trials. Clin Breast Cancer. 2018;18(5):e825–40.
21. Skiba-Tatarska M, et al. The side-effects of head and neck tumors radiotherapy. Pol Merkur Lekarski. 2016;41(241):47–9.
22. Hufnagle JJ, Goyal A. Radiation therapy induced cardiac toxicity. In StatPearls. 2020: Treasure Island (FL).
23. Kim CJ, et al. Risk of non-Hodgkin lymphoma after radiotherapy for solid cancers. Leuk Lymphoma. 2013;54(8):1691–7.
24. Bridge P, et al. The development and evaluation of a virtual radiotherapy treatment machine using an immersive visualisation environment. Comput Educ. 2007;49(2):481–94.
25. Vertual. PEARL. 2020 [Accessed: June 7, 2020]; Available from: https://www.vertual.co.uk/products/pearl/.
26. Jimenez YA, Lewis SJ. Radiation therapy patient education review and a case study using the virtual environment for radiotherapy training system. J Med Imaging Radiat Sci. 2018;49(1):106–17.

27. Zafar SY, et al. The financial toxicity of cancer treatment: a pilot study assessing out-of-pocket expenses and the insured cancer patient's experience. Oncologist. 2013;18(4):381–90.
28. Murphy CC, et al. Polypharmacy and patterns of prescription medication use among cancer survivors. Cancer. 2018;124(13):2850–7.
29. Kelley RK, Venook AP. Nonadherence to imatinib during an economic downturn. N Engl J Med. 2010;363(6):596–8.
30. Sedjo RL, Devine S. Predictors of non-adherence to aromatase inhibitors among commercially insured women with breast cancer. Breast Cancer Res Treat. 2011;125(1):191–200.
31. Lentz R, Benson AB 3rd, Kircher S. Financial toxicity in cancer care: prevalence, causes, consequences, and reduction strategies. J Surg Oncol. 2019;120(1):85–92.
32. Finkelstein EA, et al. The personal financial burden of cancer for the working-aged population. Am J Manag Care. 2009;15(11):801–6.
33. Ramsey S, et al. Washington state cancer patients found to be at greater risk for bankruptcy than people without a cancer diagnosis. Health Aff (Millwood). 2013;32(6):1143–52.
34. Zafar SY, et al. Population-based assessment of cancer survivors' financial burden and quality of life: a prospective cohort study. J Oncol Pract. 2015;11(2):145–50.
35. Bestvina CM, et al. Patient-oncologist cost communication, financial distress, and medication adherence. J Oncol Pract. 2014;10(3):162–7.
36. Ferrell BR, et al. Integration of palliative care into standard oncology care: American Society of Clinical Oncology clinical practice guideline update. J Clin Oncol. 2017;35(1):96–112.
37. National Consensus Project for Quality Palliative, C. Clinical practice guidelines for quality palliative care. Kans Nurse. 2004;79(9):16–20.
38. Dy SM, Isenberg SR, Al Hamayel NA. Palliative Care for Cancer Survivors. Med Clin North Am. 2017;101(6):1181–96.
39. Smith TJ, et al. American Society of Clinical Oncology provisional clinical opinion: the integration of palliative care into standard oncology care. J Clin Oncol. 2012;30(8):880–7.
40. Cherny N, et al. European Society for Medical Oncology (ESMO) program for the integration of oncology and palliative care: a 5-year review of the designated Centers' incentive program. Ann Oncol. 2010;21(2):362–9.
41. Dans M, et al. NCCN guidelines insights: palliative care, version 2.2017. J Natl Compr Cancer Netw. 2017;15(8):989–97.
42. Davis MP, Gutgsell T, Gamier P. What is the difference between palliative care and hospice care? Cleve Clin J Med. 2015;82(9):569–71.
43. Wright AA, et al. Associations between end-of-life discussions, patient mental health, medical care near death, and caregiver bereavement adjustment. JAMA. 2008;300(14):1665–73.
44. Wright AA, et al. Family perspectives on aggressive cancer care near the end of life. JAMA. 2016;315(3):284–92.
45. Wright AA, et al. Place of death: correlations with quality of life of patients with cancer and predictors of bereaved caregivers' mental health. J Clin Oncol. 2010;28(29):4457–64.
46. Ornstein KA, et al. Association between hospice use and depressive symptoms in surviving spouses. JAMA Intern Med. 2015;175(7):1138–46.
47. Kumar P, et al. Family perspectives on hospice care experiences of patients with cancer. J Clin Oncol. 2017;35(4):432–9.
48. Van Cutsem E, Arends J. The causes and consequences of cancer-associated malnutrition. Eur J Oncol Nurs. 2005;9(Suppl 2):S51–63.
49. Arends J, et al. ESPEN guidelines on nutrition in cancer patients. Clin Nutr. 2017;36(1):11–48.
50. Duran-Poveda M, et al. Integral nutritional approach to the care of cancer patients: results from a Delphi panel. Clin Transl Oncol. 2018;20(9):1202–11.
51. Prado CM, et al. Central tenet of cancer cachexia therapy: do patients with advanced cancer have exploitable anabolic potential? Am J Clin Nutr. 2013;98(4):1012–9.
52. Bozzetti F, et al. ESPEN guidelines on parenteral nutrition: non-surgical oncology. Clin Nutr. 2009;28(4):445–54.

53. Paccagnella A, Morassutti I, Rosti G. Nutritional intervention for improving treatment tolerance in cancer patients. Curr Opin Oncol. 2011;23(4):322–30.
54. Arends J, et al. ESPEN guidelines on enteral nutrition: non-surgical oncology. Clin Nutr. 2006;25(2):245–59.
55. August DA, et al. A.S.P.E.N. clinical guidelines: nutrition support therapy during adult anticancer treatment and in hematopoietic cell transplantation. JPEN J Parenter Enteral Nutr. 2009;33(5):472–500.
56. French Speaking Society of Clinical, N. and Metabolism. Clinical nutrition guidelines of the French Speaking Society of Clinical Nutrition and Metabolism (SFNEP): summary of recommendations for adults undergoing non-surgical anticancer treatment. Dig Liver Dis. 2014;46(8):667–74.
57. Balogh EP, et al. Patient-centered cancer treatment planning: improving the quality of oncology care. Summary of an Institute of Medicine workshop. Oncologist. 2011;16(12):1800–5.
58. Borneman T, Ferrell B, Puchalski CM. Evaluation of the FICA tool for spiritual assessment. J Pain Symptom Manag. 2010;40(2):163–73.
59. Puchalski CM. The FICA spiritual history tool #274. J Palliat Med. 2014;17(1):105–6.
60. Astrow AB, et al. Spiritual needs and perception of quality of care and satisfaction with care in hematology/medical oncology patients: a multicultural assessment. J Pain Symptom Manag. 2018;55(1):56–64.e1.
61. Lazenby M. Understanding and addressing the religious and spiritual needs of advanced cancer patients. Semin Oncol Nurs. 2018;34(3):274–83.
62. Breitbart W, et al. Meaning-centered group psychotherapy: an effective intervention for improving psychological well-being in patients with advanced cancer. J Clin Oncol. 2015;33(7):749–54.
63. Ando M, et al. Factors in narratives to questions in the short-term life review interviews of terminally ill cancer patients and utility of the questions. Palliat Support Care. 2012;10(2):83–90.
64. Guo Q, et al. Development and evaluation of the dignity talk question framework for palliative patients and their families: a mixed-methods study. Palliat Med. 2018;32(1):195–205.

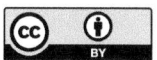

Chapter 16
Data Unit, Translational Research, and Registries

Fazal Hussain, Saud Alhayli, and Mahmoud Aljurf

Research is the core competency and the third most crucial pillar of any major cancer center, followed by patient care and teaching. Research and development is a dynamic process with a myriad of dimensions, applications, and deliverables as the backbone of evidence-based medicine. If planned and executed correctly, it can yield huge dividends as per the center's mission, vision, and lines of effort. Establishing a center of excellence to deliver world-class medicine is the patients' right and the state's obligation. Collaborative research with locoregional and international partners to offer the most advanced cancer care with dignity, respect, and the best possible QOL is noble. Challenging the existing standards of care and continuously improving cancer care is the silver lining of research. Cancer research has morphed into a tremendously relevant role for more comprehensive and long-term approaches. Shifting the paradigm, achieving new pinnacles by administering most innovative and novel therapies, devices, interventions, and techniques remain the primary objective of research for improving survival outcomes. Clinical research has witnessed unprecedented growth in recent years and has emerged as an area of high priority. Health improvement and optimization is directly linked to global security. The robust leadership, culture of research, continuous quality improvement, and research infrastructure are the cornerstones of the most efficient cancer care for measurable and quantifiable outcomes [1].

F. Hussain (✉)
College of Medicine, Alfaisal University, Riyadh, Saudi Arabia
e-mail: fhussain@alfaisal.edu

S. Alhayli · M. Aljurf
Oncology Center, King Faisal Specialist Hospital & Research Centre, Riyadh, Saudi Arabia
e-mail: salhayli@kfshrc.edu.sa; maljurf@kfshrc.edu.sa

Research Data Unit

The research unit serves as an institutional hub for initiation and registration of clinical trials by the clinicians/investigators, monitoring accrual to each protocol, budget negotiation, clinical trial agreements for research trials, and developing SOPS to facilitate centralized management of clinical studies. The research unit aims at providing the best possible quality care and a wide array of investigational therapeutic options to patients with highly advanced cancers, which would not be available otherwise. A well-structured research unit can be of immense help in streamlining and increasing efficiency for quantifiable and measurable outcomes. It is well-positioned for patient safety, higher recruitment and retention rates, quality data, and reduced study timelines and costs. The most commonly used staffing models in the research unit are team-based model (individual PIs head separate research team) and a more traditional centralized model (research supervisors assign research and support staff from pooled department resources to individual PI for each project). Research unit manages the design, conduct, approval, and analysis of research by providing comprehensive data management support to researchers as per the IPPs for efficient, quality, and statistically sound research outcomes as follows:

- *Staffing*: Qualified and trained research staff with adequate process knowledge are pivotal for data management, multidisciplinary coordination, biological specimen processing/handling, and managing regulatory issues. Research staff is responsible for designing Case Report Forms (CRFs), documentation, database designing, data entry, data validation, discrepancy management, adverse events reporting, and data extraction. Research staff provides the support and conducive environment for the investigators and clinicians to conduct for locoregional and international clinical trials/registries/databases (from proposal inception to publication) as per the local and international standards (ICH-GCP, CIOMS, NIH OHRP, Declaration of Helsinki).
- *Data management*: Research unit supports the researchers during the entire life cycle of a clinical trial by determining patients' eligibility, screening, workup, informed consent process, randomization, follow-up, protocol-specific procedure as per the timelines, data entry, regulatory compliance, pharmacy coordination, quality assurance, risk communication/reporting, document submission, and management for enrolled patients of research protocols. Data accuracy, reliability, and consistency are the minimum essential requirements for quality research programs. A wide variety of data management e-tools are being used to efficiently capture, store, and process tremendous amounts of data from multiple sources in one central platform for high-quality output. The most used commercial software are RAVE, ORACLE CLINICAL, CLINTRIAL, MACRO, and eClinical Suite as per the Code of Federal Regulations (CFR), 21 CFR Part 11. Some of the open-source software are TrialDB, openCDMS, OpenClinica, and PhOSCo. SOPs and control measures of the research unit ensure the integrity, confidentiality, and authenticity of research data.

- *Regulatory compliance*: The roles and responsibilities of the research unit include the development and implementation of research protocols, administrative support, regulatory support, monitoring subject accrual, and providing support for institutional leadership. Supporting clinical/translational review committees, data and safety monitoring committee, and QA committees in addition to continuing education and training for research staff are done by the research unit. Regulatory compliance is pivotal for generating high-quality data for an accurate trial outcome.
- *Investigational drug management/pharmacovigilance*: Research unit provides effective stakeholder coordination for study-specific drug shipment, dispensing, and administration as per protocol. Adverse drug reaction reporting, pharmacovigilance, risk management, and patient safety are critical elements of clinical research and are addressed, monitored, coordinated by the research unit through effective communication and robust teamwork. Patient safety monitoring during research studies is a critical component throughout the conduct of the study and requires effective and timely communication among all the stakeholders.
- *Quality assurance*: It is the fundamental process for generating high-quality, accurate, reliable, complete, and suitable data for statistical analysis as per protocol parameters and requirements. QA is the best way to determine protocol deviations and noncompliance. Quality data have minimal unknown or missing variables and acceptable level of protocol deviations in accordance with regulatory requirements specified for data quality. Periodic QA site visits and audits are conducted by the sponsors for protocol compliance. Institutions also have built-in internal and external audit programs for continuous quality improvement.

Translational Research (TR)

TR encompasses multidisciplinary and multidirectional coordination of laboratory and clinical research to enhance disease control and improve survival. The purpose of this bench to bedside approach is to facilitate the application of newly acquired knowledge to the patient, effectively and expeditiously, to maximize the benefit, minimum adverse events, and optimize the treatment outcomes. Translational research is the application of laboratory research innovations through preclinical studies to the patients in the clinic through clinical trials with agility to improve health outcomes. Translational research can be divided into three domains: From bench to bedside; from bench to public health; and industrialization of medical research processes. TR requires very close collaboration between the clinicians and the scientists through effective teamwork and communication. Continuous funding helps maintain the infrastructure and the minimum essential manning for the research facilities. Quality management is a pivotal part of the translational research.

Paradigmatically contextualized within the emerging purview of oncology research, translational research has become a vital tenet of accelerating research into complex cancer treatments that conflate a balance between costs of administration, primary effectiveness, and adverse implications on patient well-being. Axiomatic translational research entails the creation of an unimpeded continuum of clinical dynamics which encapsulate both clinical and basic research. The purview of collaboration rectifies the capacity for clinicians to accelerate the transition from bench to bedside. The insidious implications of ineffective collaboration are amplified amongst singular basic research institutions whose activity is contingent on the clinical care conducted by surrounding institutions, ensuring a streamlined approach to collecting adequate data samples measuring drug efficacy. Further establishment of lines of communication between all constituent actors involved across the research continuum facilitates the rigorous testing required to ensure the viability of potential cancer medications, cultivating long-term prospects for the most effective remedial practices. Stagnated collaboration has the potential to instigate debilitating parameters for further innovative oncological research not conducive to the rapid conditions required to venture into all ostensible treatments. Collaboration, however, entails robust leadership with an emphasis on the creation of standardized quality guidelines across all disciplines embedded within the mechanism of translational research. Standardized guidelines, pertaining to clinical follow-ups and procedural methods, would ensure mitigation of potential discontinuities arising across the interdisciplinary, diverse translational research team. Furthermore, standardized guidelines for translational research would essentially streamline all subsequent trials, preventing the need to pursue trial and error strategies for clinical implementation of research practices.

The equitable dissemination of research-related expertise, resources, and technical knowledge would ameliorate more efficient research processes, thus potentially facilitating an increased capacity for diverse research activity simultaneously. Concurrent mechanisms, notably the demand for a streamlined accessibility of foundational resources to facilitate the unimpeded transition from bench to bedside, is elemental in reconciling the gap along the continuum of research and preventing the stagnation of novel research. Funding allocated towards the fields of data transfer for the dissemination of information characterizes the remainder of clinical testing subsequent to embracing its transition from the bedside, shifting crucial information from clinical results to the preclinical investigator who seeks to discern any potential adverse outcomes from the experimental treatment.

Registry

One of the most efficient instruments of data management is disease-specific registries to generate high-quality, reliable, and statistically sound data. These registries, frequently referred to as outcomes registries, are "organized systems" that use observational study methods to collect uniform data. Specified outcomes are evaluated by the disease-specific registries for predetermined clinical, scientific, and administrative end state. Currently, myriads of local, national, regional, and international registries exist to collect information about cancer outcomes. These registries have played a pivotal role in determining trends, patterns, treatment practices, toxicities, patterns of failures, and survival outcomes.

Wide array of registries exist, globally, each with a well-defined and specific aims and objectives. These registries are managed by academic institutions, cooperative groups, professional organizations, third parties, public and private authorities, or researchers. Registries vary in the type, depth, timeline, and outcome variables. Overtime registries are evolving to complement and collaborate with each other to provide even larger pool of data to expand future joint research activities. A critical development in the last few years has been the recommendations by the World Health Organization (WHO) that data capturing and outcome analysis needs to be essential element of treatment and mandatory instead of an option for transplant centers. This chapter will focus on establishing an effective prospective institutional database with a silver lining in ensuring data quality and functions of HSCT registries by highlighting the processes involved and tools and standards adopted along with the roles and responsibilities of the team members. It will further highlight the challenges faced in reporting to international outcome registries, including CIBMTR, EBMT, and others.

Registry Fundamentals Observational data is highly valuable research tool in assessing utilization and patterns of medical care as well as facilitating outcomes analysis to fill evidence gaps regarding safety and effectiveness. Patient registries, typically referred to as outcomes registries, are the "organized systems" that utilize observational study methods to collect uniform data to assess predetermined outcomes for a particular exposure or disease. Highly valuable registry output serves as the rationale for future scientific and clinical trials or policy purposes [2]. Registries can be classified according to how their populations are defined and their objectives. Populations may be defined according to disease or conditions, exposures such disease managements, interventions, or side effects, or other variables like socioeconomic status. Registries are most used to capture demographics, exposures, or natural history of disease, treatment efficacy, safety, complications, adverse events, quality of life, and changing patterns of disease in an organized manner.

Registries facilitate research by addressing questions difficult to answer by clinical trials [3] or complementing clinical trial findings [4]. If data collection is sufficiently comprehensive, outcome analysis from registries could be broadly generalizable. Registries can be pivotal in continuous quality improvement, maximizing patient care, and reducing complications by reporting loops and data feedback.

Registries based upon international ethical and quality standards are considered of high scientific value for outcome analysis. Easy accessibility, credibility, accuracy, integrity, and confidentiality are the essential ingredients of a quality registry. Registries can promote research in the region, identify locoregional trends and practices, standards, and interventions, and may also be helpful in benchmarking disease outcomes. Comparison with European Group for Blood and Marrow Transplantation (EBMT) registry has shown that national registries can be used to benchmark outcome using the EBMT registry as reference [5]. The Center for International Blood and Marrow Transplantation (CIBMTR) assesses yearly survival after allogeneic HSCTs in each of the US transplant centers for participating centers and the public [6, 7]. Globalization of HSCT donor and patient registration is a realistic goal and could lead to donor safety, better treatments, and outcomes [8, 9]. Registry data have provided important insights into international differences in indications for HSCT, and access to HSCT [10]. Data from outcome registries is helpful for comparative analysis to further refine therapeutic intervention and improve outcomes. Outcome registries face a myriad of challenges and are summarized as follows:

Research Personnel Adequately qualified and properly trained research professionals with sound medical background and experience with multidisciplinary approach are essential. Critical experts in the operation of the registry include clinical/scientific, project management, biostatistics and epidemiology, data managers, database administrators, regulatory compliance, and expertise in quality assurance. Staff familiarization with basic principles of cancer epidemiology, terminology, therapeutic interventions, and outcomes can substantially increase the value of registry. Cohesive teamwork is the key for optimizing the value of the registry throughout the registry life cycle by data capturing, analysis, dissemination, reporting, and publications.

Regulations – Managing Ethical, Privacy, and Legal Considerations Maintaining privacy and confidentiality, protection of human subjects and legal issues in data management (ownership, collection, and data exchange) are the major tenets of registry. Robust security mechanisms are crucial to safeguards the rights of registry participants, especially for the registry involving international collaboration. The bylaws, data transfer agreements, accreditation for standardization are pivotal in streamlining regulatory trepidations. However, wide-ranging variations in IRB regulations and cultural sensitivities can be challenging, especially for multinational registries. However, because outcomes registries are observational, they are often considered "low risk" with regard to the potential for harm to human subjects. The registry must address consent for the use of data for research obtained from research subjects by outcomes registries; however, registry functions for public health or government program purposes may not require specific consent for research [11].

Data Management Scope and quality of data determines the usefulness of a registry. The scope of the data collected is framed by purpose and objectives and is influenced by myriad factors (geographic location, setting of data collection, cost). The size of the registry can vary depending upon the number of observations required to achieve the desired end states.

Registries have well-defined core dataset of essential data elements and patient outcomes as per the purpose and objectives. Core data sets and CRFs are reviewed and revised periodically to align with evolving diagnostic, therapeutic and prognostic markers. Accuracy, integrity, and data completeness are the most critical elements in the quality and value of a registry. Most data collection for HSCT outcomes registries is conducted using electronic applications. Sound quality information systems are needed for effective data collection to support the registry.

Cultural Sensitivities and Communication Issues Particularly, international registries are managed by continuous education and training in a unified manner to overcome tremendous cultural, social, and economic heterogeneity. Culturally sensitive tools (QOL form, etc.) can help enhance registry compliance.

Performance/Quality Management Registry (e.g., HSCT) can be a crucial component of a center's quality management/performance improvement programs. The accreditation bodies for HSCT in the US and Europe (FACT, ISCT, EBMT-JACIE, etc.) mandate that transplant centers collect and utilize standard core dataset defined by the field to analyze and understand their program quality [12]. Accreditation helps in implementing basic unified standards for good clinical practice among all participating centers for accuracy, integrity, and transparency of registry data. Outcomes registries can also provide a quality context or benchmark for HSCT centers when evaluating their program's performance. Quality management research can also be facilitated by outcome registries, which can lead to better survival outcomes by improving transplant practices. Registries facilitates uniformity in lab standards, toxicity criteria (Bearman) [13],GVHD definitions (National Institutes of Health [NIH] [14], and performance status (Karnofsky Performance Status [KPS], Eastern Cooperative Oncology Group [ECOG]/Zubrod, etc.). High-quality registry encompasses advanced methodology, operational excellence, enhanced validity, and discernible outcomes.

Data Utilization and Publications Observational research findings yield in significant clinical improvement and clinical trial planning [15]. Data sharing and collaborative research for optimizing patient outcomes is the key to a useful registry [16–17]. Many cancer centers report their data to comprehensive global registries (CIBMTR, EBMT, etc.). Interoperability, interfacing, and integration can maximize outcome and utility of these registries. Well-outlined and clear authorship guidelines are followed and unanimously approved by the participating centers based upon the number of patients, intellectual contributions, and center participation. Registry enhances the understanding of disease outcomes by addressing key questions like intervention results in specific patient groups, prognostic factors, new therapeutic regimens, comparison of therapies, inter-center practice, and outcome variability, capturing delayed adverse events and novel analytic approaches [18].

Registry can help in determining the efficacy of innovative and novel therapeutic strategies, assess outcomes, accrual patterns, generalizability, and patient selection practices. Registries can provide valuable data for well-designed retrospective observational studies to improve clinical practice [19–21]and plan future clinical trials [22].

Funding and Sustainability Registry operations to collect complete, high-quality data are resource-intense and funding-dependent. Sponsors include government agencies, scientific grant organizations, research collaborators, pharmaceutical manufacturers, accreditation bodies, philanthropic organizations, and others. Funding could be for the overall operations of the registry or a specific research project. Some sponsors may have vested interest, and partially fund the registry, for capturing the utilization data of a particular product, device, or intervention.

Outcomes registries must remain vigilant for an innovation or collaborative opportunities to use or expand the registry to seize new funding opportunities.

Conclusion

There is a growing need to develop high-quality research infrastructure in newly developing cancer centers. Existing international models are a great resource for adopting best practices in establishing the research unit with advanced capabilities and procedures for data capturing, data quality monitoring, data analysis, strategic communication, and publications. Well-positioned, fully operational and optimally functional research unit should be able to provide highly valuable information and data that would not be available otherwise. The data quality standardization is vital to determine the scientific credibility and reliability of a research entity. A critical development in the last few years has been the recommendation of the World Health Organization (WHO) to make the data collection and analysis an integral part of the therapy rather than a choice for cancer programs.

References

1. Tang C, Hess KR, Sanders D, et al. Modifying the clinical research infrastructure at a dedicated clinical trials unit: assessment of trial development, activation, and participant accrual. Clin Cancer Res. 2017;23(6):1407–13. https://doi.org/10.1158/1078-0432.CCR-16-1936.
2. Gliklich RE, Dreyer NA, editors. Registries for evaluating patient outcomes: a user's guide. 2nd ed. (Prepared by Outcome DEcIDE Center [Outcome Sciences, Inc. d/b/a Outcome] under Contract No. HHSA290200500351 TO3.) AHRQ Publication No. 10-EHC049. Rockville, MD: Agency for Healthcare Research and Quality, September 2010.
3. Horowitz M. The role of registries in facilitating clinical research in BMT: examples from the Center for International Blood and Marrow Transplant Research. Bone Marrow Transplant. 2008;42(Suppl 1):S1–2. https://doi.org/10.1038/bmt.2008.101.
4. Horowitz MM, Przepiorka D, Bartels P, et al. Tacrolimus vs. cyclosporine immunosuppression: results in advanced-stage disease compared with historical controls treated exclusively with cyclosporine. Biol Blood Marrow Transplant. 1999;5(3):180–6. https://doi.org/10.1053/bbmt.1999.v5.pm10392964.
5. Russell NH, Szydlo R, McCann S, et al. The use of a national transplant registry to benchmark transplant outcome for patients undergoing autologous and allogeneic stem cell transplantation in the United Kingdom and Ireland. Br J Haematol. 2004;124(4):499–503. https://doi.org/10.1046/j.1365-2141.2003.04793.x.
6. http://bethematch.org. For-Patients and Families/Getting a transplant/Choosing a transplant centre/US transplant centres. Last accessed 31 May, 2020.
7. http://www.cibmtr.org/Meetings/Materials/CSOAForum/Pages/index.aspx. CIBMTR Center-Specific Outcomes Analysis. Last accessed 28 May, 2020.
8. Kodera Y. The Japan marrow donor program, the Japan cord blood Bank network and the Asia blood and marrow transplant registry. Bone Marrow Transplant. 2008;42(Suppl 1):S6. https://doi.org/10.1038/bmt.2008.103.
9. Atsuta Y, Suzuki R, Yoshimi A, et al. Unification of hematopoietic stem cell transplantation registries in Japan and establishment of the TRUMP system. Int J Hematol. 2007;86(3):269–74. https://doi.org/10.1532/IJH97.06239.

10. Gratwohl A, Baldomero H, Aljurf M, et al. Hematopoietic stem cell transplantation: a global perspective. JAMA. 2010;303(16):1617–24. https://doi.org/10.1001/jama.2010.491.
11. http://www.hhs.gov/ocr/privacy/hipaa/understanding/special/publichealth/.   Health Information Privacy and Public Health, US Department of Health and Human Services. Last accessed 1 June, 2020.
12. http://www.factwebsite.org/uploadedFiles/FACT_News/Final%20Draft%205th%20 Edition%20Accreditation%20Manual.04.18.11.pdf. FACT-JACIE International Standards for Cellular Therapy Product Collection, Processing, and Administration, Fourth Edition. Last accessed 30 May, 2020.
13. Bearman SI, Appelbaum FR, Buckner CD, et al. Regimen-related toxicity in patients undergoing bone marrow transplantation. J Clin Oncol. 1988;6(10):1562–8. https://doi.org/10.1200/JCO.1988.6.10.1562.
14. Filipovich AH, Weisdorf D, Pavletic S, et al. National Institutes of Health consensus development project on criteria for clinical trials in chronic graft-versus-host disease: I. Diagnosis and staging working group report. Biol Blood Marrow Transplant. 2005;11(12):945–56. https://doi.org/10.1016/j.bbmt.2005.09.004.
15. Pasquini MC, Griffith LM, Arnold DL, et al. Hematopoietic stem cell transplantation for multiple sclerosis: collaboration of the CIBMTR and EBMT to facilitate international clinical studies. Biol Blood Marrow Transplant. 2010;16(8):1076–83. https://doi.org/10.1016/j.bbmt.2010.03.012.
16. Locatelli F, Crotta A, Ruggeri A, et al. Analysis of risk factors influencing outcomes after cord blood transplantation in children with juvenile myelomonocytic leukemia: a EUROCORD, EBMT, EWOG-MDS, CIBMTR study. Blood. 2013;122(12):2135–41. https://doi.org/10.1182/blood-2013-03-491589.
17. Ruggeri A, Eapen M, Scaravadou A, et al. Umbilical cord blood transplantation for children with thalassemia and sickle cell disease. Biol Blood Marrow Transplant. 2011;17(9):1375–82. https://doi.org/10.1016/j.bbmt.2011.01.012.
18. Rizzo JD, Curtis RE, Socié G, et al. Solid cancers after allogeneic hematopoietic cell transplantation. Blood. 2009;113(5):1175–83. https://doi.org/10.1182/blood-2008-05-158782.
19. Anderlini P, Rizzo JD, Nugent ML, et al. Peripheral blood stem cell donation: an analysis from the International Bone Marrow Transplant Registry (IBMTR) and European Group for Blood and Marrow Transplant (EBMT) databases. Bone Marrow Transplant. 2001;27(7):689–92. https://doi.org/10.1038/sj.bmt.1702875.
20. Lee SJ, Storer B, Wang H, et al. Providing personalized prognostic information for adult leukemia survivors. Biol Blood Marrow Transplant. 2013;19(11):1600–7. https://doi.org/10.1016/j.bbmt.2013.08.013.
21. Eapen M, Klein JP, Ruggeri A, et al. Impact of allele-level HLA matching on outcomes after myeloablative single unit umbilical cord blood transplantation for hematologic malignancy. Blood. 2014;123(1):133–40.
22. Jacobsohn DA, Arora M, Klein JP, et al. Risk factors associated with increased nonrelapse mortality and with poor overall survival in children with chronic graft-versus-host disease. Blood. 2011;118(16):4472–9. https://doi.org/10.1182/blood-2011-04-349068.

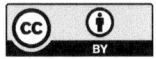

Chapter 17
Education and Training

Hemant S. Murthy, Rami Manochakian, and Mohamed A. Kharfan-Dabaja

Introduction

One of the main missions of any comprehensive cancer center is to provide opportunities for training and education to improve prevention and treatment outcomes of cancer patients. Management of cancer in today's era is multidisciplinary, with patient care teams comprised of multispecialty physicians, advanced practice providers (APPs), nurses, therapists, and other health-care staff across different fields. Each team member holds a specific role in cancer care and has a different approach to the management of patients ultimately leading to more comprehensive care.

Given the many components and specialties that comprise a comprehensive cancer center, the educational programs are often specialized and tailored to multiple disciplines. The ultimate goal of establishing education and training programs within a comprehensive cancer center is not only to have them available to their staff, but rather to garner the ability to disseminate education to health-care providers, cancer patients, and the public at large.

Training of Health-Care Professionals

Within a cancer center, there is a variety of specialties which provide expertise in oncology. These specialties possess their own individual training programs that help train and develop future physicians, scientists, APPs, and nurses specialized within

H. S. Murthy · M. A. Kharfan-Dabaja (✉)
Division of Hematology-Oncology, Mayo Clinic, Jacksonville, FL, USA

Blood and Marrow Transplantation Program, Mayo Clinic, Jacksonville, FL, USA
e-mail: KharfanDabaja.Mohamed@mayo.edu

R. Manochakian
Division of Hematology-Oncology, Mayo Clinic, Jacksonville, FL, USA

© The Author(s) 2022
M. Aljurf et al. (eds.), *The Comprehensive Cancer Center*,
https://doi.org/10.1007/978-3-030-82052-7_17

oncology. Training programs may include but are not limited to biomedical and basic science research, postdoctoral programs, clinical residency and/or fellowship programs, all geared towards research and treatment of cancer.

Hematology/Medical Oncology

Hematologists and medical oncologists comprise the largest block of cancer specialists in a comprehensive cancer center. Their standard training is called "Hematology/Oncology fellowship", which in the USA follows completion of 3 years of internal medicine residency, but that is not always the case in other countries. A hematology/oncology fellowship typically requires 3 years, although some programs offer the opportunity for a 2-year fellowship in either hematology or medical oncology. The goal of fellowship training programs is to enable trainees to gain a broad knowledge of clinical and research cancer sciences, and to develop the needed clinical skills and expertise to become competent and proficient hematologists and/or oncologists. At least half of the fellowship curriculum is spent in clinical training with a combination of inpatient and outpatient experiences, focusing on different malignancies including solid tumors, benign hematology, malignant hematology, and hematopoietic cell transplantation (HCT) or other cellular therapies. Many programs offer dedicated research time that can be spent in basic science or in clinical/observational investigation, depending on the trainees' interest and it is usually under the guidance and tutelage of a research mentor. Trainees present their research projects at national scientific meetings and ultimately publish the findings in peer-reviewed journals.

Apart from clinical training and research, another major component of a fellowship program is the didactic and experiential learning lectures and activities, which are embedded within the context of health-care delivery system. It also provides trainees with access to comprehensive education resources provided by major national hematology and oncology societies, namely, the American Society of Clinical Oncology (ASCO), the American Society of Hematology (ASH), and others. Some centers offer an additional 1 year of subspecialty cancer training after completion of the 3 years fellowship, like fellowships in leukemia, blood and marrow transplantation, thoracic malignancies and others, or in drug development and early cancer therapeutics trials.

Pediatric Hematology/Medical Oncology

A pediatric hematology/oncology fellowship curriculum also requires 3 years and mirrors that of the medical oncology/hematology fellowship.

Radiation Oncology

One field that differs slightly in this training model is radiation oncology. In the USA, radiation oncology is a 5 year residency program for which candidates may apply for and join directly out of medical school. The first year is generally a transitional year of a medical internship followed by 4 years of radiation oncology training. Radiation oncology residency training prepares for treatment of both adult and pediatric populations and most of the training occurs in the outpatient setting. Time for research is also embedded in many radiation oncology programs.

Other Oncology Specialties

Oncology specialty training also includes surgical oncology and gynecology oncology. Similar to medical and pediatric oncology programs, eligible trainees must have completed residencies in their respective fields before pursuing oncology specialty training. The length of residency and fellowship training may vary. We refer the reader to the Accreditation Council of Graduate Medical Education oncology specialty training programs for additional details (https://www.acgme.org).

Pharmacy

Pharmacists with specific expertise in oncology often go through additional training, including attaining board certification in oncology pharmacy (BCOP) [1]. BCOP is a credential for pharmacists whose practice involve understanding the complexity of drug therapies use for preventing and treating cancer, manage cancer-related and drug-related adverse events, or clinical situations not encountered in other diseases. To obtain BCOP, they are required to graduate from an accredited pharmacy program, followed by completion of a 2 year pharmacy residency program, which includes 1 year dedicated to oncology pharmacy training followed by passing score on standardized board certification examination.

Basic Science/Laboratory Researcher

The Cancer Biology Training Consortium (CABTRAC) was created in 2005 in order to help develop and facilitate training recommendations for future cancer researchers, especially graduate and postgraduate researchers [2]. The goal of CABTRAC was to establish guidelines for trainees focused on education in the experimental science of cancer biology, research training in the experimental science of cancer biology, and career development of trainees towards independent cancer biologists [3]. Trainees are expected to be exposed to topics including basic science of cancer biology: dysregulation of signal transduction pathways, oncogenes and tumor suppressor genes, control of cell proliferation, cell cycle, and cell death, carcinogenesis, DNA damage, and repair, tumor angiogenesis, invasion, and metastases, tumor microenvironment, cancer genetics and epigenetics, cancer immunology, translational science (molecular diagnosis and prognosis, molecular imaging, systems biology and bioinformatics, therapeutic strategies including targeted and cytotoxic therapies, immunotherapy, hormone therapy, small molecules), and chemoprevention. Educational exposure to biostatistics, informatics, data interpretation, cancer disparities, and basic experimental design is also deemed essential to the training of cancer biology scientists.

Continued Medical Education (CME)

Training and education in a comprehensive cancer center are not restricted to trainees within a structured training program. Continued education of all cancer care team members is essential, given the always changing understanding of cancer biology and emergence of new therapies, technologies, and innovations. The goals of CME as it pertains to members of a cancer center are twofold: to enhance their knowledge and skills pertaining to their own individual practices and specialties and acquiring knowledge from other specialties (also known as cross-training). Some examples of cross-training include incorporating novel concepts that can be investigated across multiple diseases, or awareness of clinical scenarios that may allow lab or translational researchers to gain better insight into the cancer.

Grand Rounds

Cancer center grand rounds are regularly scheduled seminar series through which invited speakers present insights and expertise on cancer treatment and/or new innovations in cancer research. Speakers typically include cancer center members or outside invited speakers. Grand rounds can serve multiple purposes within a cancer center. It can provide members with updates in patient care and management and could be a CME source. Additionally, grand rounds, through presentation of new innovations and research findings, can also spawn collaboration and promote cross-training among specialists from different disciplines within oncology, potentially stimulating new research.

Board Certification

Many oncology specialties have board certification requirements as dictated by their respective specialty organizations. In addition, certification is often contingent on passing specialty board examinations. Maintaining board certification also requires maintaining standards including participation in educational programs, continued professional development, and satisfactorily passing board examinations. Maintenance of such standards by cancer center members is important to ensure continued training and education, remaining current with advances in oncology, and ultimately improving delivery of care to cancer patients.

Development of New Cancer-Specific Programs

Continued advancement in oncology therapeutics can sometimes be limited by expansion of these therapies to centers with limited resources. New programs are developed in order to provide education on emerging or complex therapies such as phase 1 clinical research units, HCT, and other cellular therapies.

Building specialized cancer-specific programs may be burdensome, particularly in low- to middle-income countries. Accordingly, partnering with more established cancer institutions with requisite expertise can prove beneficial. One successful example of this was the partnership of the Global BMT program of the University of Illinois at Chicago (UIC) [4] and its partnership with developing a bone marrow transplant program in Kathmandu, Nepal [5]. The steps involved included training relevant staff in Nepal and allowing for Nepalese providers to receive training at UIC, exchange of standard operating procedures, overseeing construction of HCT unit in a Nepalese hospital, and continued teleconferences between UIC and Nepal. Another example includes enhancing cancer care in low-income limited resource countries such as Guatemala, Vietnam, and Rwanda [6]. Through partnership with established cancer centers and with significant investment, improvements, and development of infrastructure, training of relevant professionals, implementing new cancer screening programs, and developing cancer-specific health policy have improved cancer care in these regions. These serve as examples of the benefits of partnering with established cancer centers with requisite experience to facilitate the development of new cancer-specific programs.

Discussion

Cancer is a major public health problem worldwide. Recent advances in the under-standing of the biologic and molecular aspect of cancer, and emergence of new and more effective targeted therapies highlight the importance of continuous education of health-care providers and supporting staff. The ultimate goal is to deliver effective treatment in a safe manner. Unfortunately, there is a gap in the ability to make these therapies and new technologies available to all cancer patients worldwide. Education and training addresses one major aspect of this problem by developing partnerships between cancer centers in the developing world and established centers in developing countries to facilitate exchange of knowledge. Regrettably, the high cost of these therapies and technologies is a serious limitation to deliver these treatments to cancer patients in the developing world.

Conflicts of Interests HSM: no conflicts of interest to disclose

RM: Discloses advisory board/consultancy for AstraZeneca, Guardant Health, Novocure and Takeda

MAK-D: Discloses consultancy for Pharmacyclics and Daiichi Sankyo

References

1. Oncology Pharmacy – Board of Pharmacy Specialties [Internet]. [cited 2020 May 22]. Available from: https://www.bpsweb.org/bps-specialties/oncology-pharmacy/.
2. Torti FM, Altieri D, Broach J, Fan H, Lotze M, Manfredi J, et al. Ph.D. training in cancer biology. Cancer Res. 2008;68(22):9122–4.
3. Welch DR, Antalis TM, Burnstein K, Vona-Davis L, Jensen RA, Nakshatri H, et al. Essential components of cancer education. Cancer Res. 2015;75(24):5202–5.
4. Olowoselu O, Amaru A, Filonenko K, Mbiine R, Tuladhar S, Rondelli D. Implementation and evaluation of the first global blood & marrow transplantation (globalbmt) training program at the university of illinois at chicago (UIC). Biol Blood Marrow Transplant. 2019;25(3):S322–3.
5. Poudyal B, Neupane S, Tuladhar S, Shrestha P, Sweiss K, Patel PR, et al. UIC Globalbmt partnered with a Government Hospital in Kathmandu to establish the first Blood & Marrow Transplant (BMT) Center in Nepal. Biol Blood Marrow Transplant. 2018;24(3):S312–3.
6. Wagner CM, Antillón F, Uwinkindi F, Thuan TV, Luna-Fineman S, Anh PT, et al. Establishing cancer treatment programs in resource-limited settings: lessons learned.

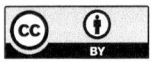

Chapter 18
Cancer Management at Sites with Limited Resources: Challenges and Potential Solutions

Shahrukh K. Hashmi, Fady Geara, Asem Mansour, and Mahmoud Aljurf

The World Bank defines low-income economies ($1005 or less GNI per capita) or lower middle-income economies ($1006 to $3955 GNI per capita) as Low- and Middle-Income Countries (LMIC) which comprise of approximately two-thirds of the world's 197 countries recognized by the United Nations.

In the LMICs, population pyramids are changing dynamically towards a constrictive pattern from an expansive pattern as the lifetime expectancy is increasing due to an ageing population [1]. As age is the greatest risk factor for cancers [2, 3], expectedly the incidence of cancer continues to increase dramatically in LMIC, which is also partly due to advancements in diagnostic techniques [4]. The majority of cancer cases globally now occur in LMIC, and 65% of cancer deaths worldwide occur in these countries [5].

Apart from economic factors, there are considerable differences in the geopolitical arenas of LMIC compared to many developed nations [6, 7]; therefore the

Authorship Contributions:
SKH wrote the first draft of the manuscript. All authors vouch for the accuracy and contents of the manuscript. All authors approved the final version of the draft

S. K. Hashmi (✉)
Division of Hematology, Department of Medicine, Mayo Clinic, Rochester, MN, USA

Sheikh Shakhbout Medical City, Abu Dhabi, UAE
e-mail: hashmi.shahrukh@mayo.edu

F. Geara
Naef K. Basile Cancer Institute, Department of Radiation Oncology, American University of Beirut, Beirut, Lebanon

A. Mansour
King Hussein Cancer Center, Amman, Jordan

M. Aljurf
Adult Hematology and HSCT, Oncology Center, King Faisal Specialist Hospital and Research Center, Riyadh, Saudi Arabia

© The Author(s) 2022
M. Aljurf et al. (eds.), *The Comprehensive Cancer Center*,
https://doi.org/10.1007/978-3-030-82052-7_18

challenges of providing comprehensive cancer care in the LMIC are different. Here, we will briefly summarize the current challenges that many LMICs face with respect to oncologic care, focusing on both prevention and therapeutics, with the caveat that these are general issues which may not apply to all LMICs.

Medical Services, Data, and Infrastructure

Need for Effective cancer Registries

A database or a registry of the cancer cases encompassing the type of tumor, stage, genomics, and other parameters is essential for overall cancer care for any country. This database could be a hospital-based or a population-based registry. Concept of population-based cancer registries is at least half a century old, as in 1950s, the American College of Surgeons (ACoS) implemented policies for development of hospital-based cancer registries. Sweden was the first country globally to establish a formal cancer registry for all cases diagnosed and linked the data with personal information (Swedish PIN and other variables). In 1973, The National Cancer Institute of the United States (US), through its Surveillance, Epidemiology and End Results (SEER) program established the first national cancer registry program which currently produces a variety of data (and analytics) on various aspects of cancer epidemiology [8].

Some LMICs have established cancer registries at federal level; however, the quality control mechanisms of these registries are extremely variable, and quite often data is either missing, or lags current data entry mechanisms which leads to consider delays in updating the data. Moreover, lack of long-term outcomes data would preclude accurate mortality or morbidity analysis. The need of accurate data of cancer cases in a country is imperative to develop cancer control programs and screening guidelines. Unless the burden of each cancer type and subtype is known, it is hard to allocate appropriate resources for prevention or treatment of the specific types of cancer. Additionally, there are a number of international grants or programs specifically for cancer-associated activities in LMICs; however, one needs to know the exact burden of the disease in order to apply for most of these grants. Therefore, the need for a cancer registry at national level should be a top priority of a country's healthcare policy. A state-of-the-art cancer center's hospital-based registry is insufficient to formulate future planning for cancer control, since it is limited to the patients coming to that center, and also due to the known phenomenon of patient shopping at various institutions (and second opinions), which may be more pronounced in the LMICs.

Given the importance of a nationwide cancer registry covering both urban and rural areas, as a solution, we would encourage both the governmental agencies and the institutional leadership to work together to develop policies for a mandatory cancer reporting mechanism and a national registry that would capture important variables (including outcomes data) and have resources to functionally sustain the registry in long run (technologic tools, data managers, statisticians etc.). The World Health Assembly in conjunction with World Health Organization (WHO) has passed the resolution Cancer Prevention and Control and has urged the governments to accelerate action to achieve the targets specified in the Global Action Plan and the "2030 United Nations Agenda for Sustainable Development". Establishment of effective cancer registries is an integral part of the proposed agenda by WHO.

Moreover, The World Bank's Regional Program of Cancer Registries (P163187) has proposed help in establishing population-based cancer registries to collect, analyze, and publish a regional compilation of cancer statistics. This is another avenue which can be evaluated for establishment of cancer registry at regional level.

Lack of Connectivity

Quite often, patients care is fragmented across the institutions. Some patients would receive initial consult at one institution, then laboratory work at another, and then radiology at a third institution. Not only the care is fragmented which can result in delay in both diagnosis and treatment, but also the information technology (IT) systems are not interfaced with each other thereby care is further affected. Having a unified IT system, or electronic medical record (EMR) systems that can interface with each other would make care better, and also would allow for a smooth transition of care between institutions. Another layer of approvals required for sharing information is the lack of clear cybersecurity laws for exchanging EMRs. Thus a conscious effort has to be made to clarify pathways for information exchange between institutions so that patient care is not affected.

Research Infrastructure

The improvement in the cancer survival is mainly due to tremendous investment in preclinical and clinical research by institutions (e.g., tertiary care hospitals), governmental agencies (e.g., National Institutes of Health), and the pharmaceutical industry. However, most of the innovation and discovery in oncology (including genomics and drug development) has come from investigators from the developed countries. A robust research infrastructure is required to assimilate all three phases of research, that is, basic science, translational, and clinical trials.

Basic science: The investment in preclinical research requires considerable resources that include laboratory and equipment as well as expertise [9]. Scientific collaborations with global experts is necessary at least in initial phases of setup of basic science laboratories, which require expensive equipment (and reagents) and human resources (PhD, and advanced technicians, besides postdoctoral trainees).

Clinical trials: For clinical research, the institutional leadership and the governmental agencies must invest both in infrastructure (e.g., clinical trials unit) and in human resources [10]. The phase I, II, and III clinical trials require funding as expertise, and once the infrastructure is available (including CRCs, clinical trialists, and biostatisticians), then physician-scientists would be able to produce (write up protocols and successfully accrue the projected number of subjects) results from clinical research, and moreover attract cutting-edge clinical trials from pharmaceutical and biotech industry. Typically, randomized trials (mostly phase III) change the clinical practice, and over the past few decades, successful completion of randomized trials initiated by principal investigators from developing countries has been extremely rare [11, 12]. Most common pathway of executing clinical trials in LMICs is facilitation by pharmaceutical industry, and occurrence of phase I clinical trials is hardly existent in most of the LMICs [13]. Having physician-scientists who are appreciated and given ample time and resources for research is a necessary factor for the successful execution of a clinical trial.

Translational research: Some LMICs have advanced facilities for basic science research and excellent tertiary care hospitals as well both producing some degree of scientific output. To translate the preclinical models into medical field requires direct collaboration between institutions. Unless this happens, cutting-edge innovation may not occur.

A comprehensive research infrastructure would require (apart from HR, space, and equipment), effective Institutional Review Board (IRB), Data Safety Monitoring Board (DSMB), and extensive collaborations with the regulatory agencies (e.g., a country's federal drug authority or equivalent agency). How to operationalize such an infrastructure requires a huge setup which has four essential aspects – human resources (scientists, physicians, nurses, clinical research coordinators, biostatistician, clinical nurses, pharmacists, phlebotomists) physical space (including negative pressure and positive pressure rooms), equipment (laboratory and office), and software (REDCap or other databases). This requires direct interaction with local health authorities.

Tumor Boards and Multispecialty Care

Recent data has indicated that multidisciplinary care and decisions improve outcomes of cancer patients [14]. A multidisciplinary tumor board may require expertise from radiologists, medical oncologists, radiation oncologists, surgeons, pathologists, and other specialties. This pertains more to solid cancers; however, in hematologic malignancies, molecular hematology boards have become routine to discuss the cases and diagnostic dilemmas at large cancer centers in developed countries. Emphasis should be laid in assimilation of such tumor boards for cancer subtypes in developing countries, which can also foster holistic care to a patient apart from increasing research collaborations between various clinical specialties. If multispecialty tumor boards cannot be established due to limited resources or lack of expertise, then efforts could be concentrated on scheduling regular tumor board meetings at a partner institution with a large cancer center (maybe within the same country or internationally).

Building a homogeneous multidisciplinary tumor board can indeed be very challenging at the beginning. Apart from utilizing technology to have virtual boards, one must continue to organize a team to eventually establish functional tumor boards – this would require at least a medical oncologist, radiation oncologist, surgical oncologist, radiologist, pathologist, oncology nurses, coordinators, and ideally also palliative care team as well.

Human Resources

Unavailability of Specialized, but Essential Cancer Services and Human Power Radiotherapy and Stem Cell Transplantation

There are many services that are necessary for both curative and palliative management in cancers; however, due to expertise required, technology transfer issues, equipment infrastructure, and costs, they may be unavailable in LMICs. On the top of these essential services are stem cell transplantation (SCT) [15, 16] and radiotherapy [17–19]. These two services are necessary for many cancers and may be the only potential cure, and in order to achieve this cure, many patients from LMIC may travel outside their home country for the receipt of these services. One essential element of these services is that efforts must be concentrated to start with bare minimum requirements in order to establish at least one specialized unit, for example, for radiation therapy unit in a country, it is not essential to wait for funding and expertise for carbon-ion therapy or proton beam therapy, but can start with the cobalt therapy or with traditional linear accelerators. Similarly, for SCT, it is not imperative to have a huge infrastructure for allogeneic SCTs, when a center can start with the relatively low-risk autologous SCTs. Apart from getting expertise from outside the country for a new specialized program, one has to consider capacity building and skills training for physicians and nurses within a country.

Education Infrastructure

Efforts to train physicians, nurses, and technicians for specialized care is essential. This applies directly to the fields of cancer in general, but more so to the very specialized fields, for example, radiation oncology and bone marrow transplantation. There should be concentrated effort by the institutional leadership and also by the governmental agencies who regulate the medical training programs.

Quality Management and Access to Care

Sustainability and Consistency

Sustainability and consistency in quality of cancer care is a challenge in unpredictable geopolitical circumstances and, therefore, a great degree of disparity exists in the quality level among various providers (and/or institutions). Given there is a lack of effective reporting and measurement of outcomes, we propose to have simplified metrics for objective evaluation of quality of care so that the results can be shared to identify gaps and acquire best practices.

Access to cancer Care

In many countries, access to cancer care is extremely hard due to many factors particularly due to the shortage of comprehensive services, lack of expertise, and due to economic hardships due to a lack of comprehensive national coverage. Even if there is a well-established cancer center, populations may not have the resources to reach to the specialized centers due to social and financial barriers.

A study from Cameroon indicated a 6 month delay between appearance of the first sign of cancer and seeing a healthcare provider [20]. Access to a cancer specialist is significantly delayed due to a variety of reasons in LMIC, which include (but not limited to), cultural preferences (e.g., taboo in some communities) and trust issues with medical providers or allopathic physicians (with a greater emphasis on complementary and alternative medicine therapies), financial reasons, or due to a deficiency of oncologists. This must be addressed at both institutional level and national health policy level. The governmental structure should be able to cope up with the increasing demand for treating oncologists in LMICs. Moreover, disparities in access to cancer specialists and cancer-related services (e.g., PET scans, radiation oncology facility, etc.) should be addressed. Some methods could potentially be applied to improve access, for example, targeted fundraising and donations, support group initiation, negotiating with government sponsoring of cancer programs and services, and revenue sharing programs with industry.

Influence of Political Activities: Refugee Crises and Internal Displacement

According to the UN Refugee Agency (UNHCR), at least 79.5 million people around the world have been forced to flee their homes which includes nearly 26 million refugees and 47 million internally displaced people (IDP) by 2019 [21]. This leads to additional burdens for social and healthcare-related expenditures to the countries. Not only delayed diagnosis of the refugees and IDPs can lead to increased mortality, the psychosocial issues in these people can lead to considerably increased morbidity.

There has to be a concentrated effort by the governmental agencies to evaluate the exact oncologic needs of the refugees and IDPs. Mechanisms must be established to provide both urgent care and long-term planning if the refugees and IDPs are diagnosed with cancer or received initial treatment at their home country or local city before being displaced. Many hospitals may not accept refugees for cancer care, but it is the government's responsibility to provide at least emergency oncology care to the refugees and IDPs, and these include but are not limited to spinal cord compression, hypercalcemia of malignancy, superior-vena-cava syndrome, acute leukemias (ALL, APL, AML), and high-grade lymphomas (particularly Burkitt lymphoma and large cell lymphomas).

It is critical that the international or local governmental support provided by the stakeholders focus on noncommunicable diseases as hematologic and oncologic emergencies are almost always fatal if not treated urgently.

Successful Models of Cancer Care: Sharing Best Practices

Given a multitude of differences between LMIC and developed world with respect to cancer care, especially in regard to socioeconomic status (SES) of patients, regulatory agency policies, and political climates, a potential solution to successfully implement oncologic care so that outcomes in the end users improve is to partner with countries in which successful execution of the cancer programs has already occurred. This would ideally be a concept of twinning which has prevailed in developing countries to many projects both in healthcare and other sectors. A classic example is the twinning program for the establishment of a stem cell transplant program in Bangladesh with the help of expertise at every level (architecture/design, laboratory issues, transplant physician expertise, nursing training, and others), with a hospital in Boston, Massachusetts, which has resulted in successful example of technology transfer from a developed country to LMIC.

For sharing best practices, it is not essential to have physical presence of large teams in a LMIC institution or governmental agency, and a virtual contract for telehealth could also be of help for smaller projects, for example, for tumor boards.

Nonetheless, a unified standard approach is essential for a country's success so that most successful practices which have proven to improve clinical outcomes can be shared. In this instance, it is imperative that there is one professional organization which dictates not only national guidelines but also sets up research priorities. Although this seems trivial, however, in real-world practice, there are critical challenges with respect to establishing or sustaining professional organizations. For example, in some LMIC there may be two or even three professional hematology or oncology societies, all claiming national statuses in clinical and research matters. This practice of egoistic approach based on institutional or personal prides must end, and a unified organization representing the entire nation should be established. In the USA, for instance, there is one national organization for each subspecialty, for example, ASCO for medical oncology, ASTRO for radiation oncology, and ASH for hematology. To have some control to either mandate or at least encourage one national society will lead to less dispersion of knowledge and best practices.

An ideal model to cover cancer care in all LMICs does not exist; however, various models fit into the geopolitical and economic infrastructure of a country, for example, matrix cancer centers or stand-alone centers may fit into the management paradigm of different countries.

Drug Approvals and Shortages

Drug approval processes in the LMIC vary considerably and quite often is a constantly changing process with layers of bureaucratic and political interventions. Each LMIC, like the developed countries, has a drug regulatory authority or agency; however, efficiency differs tremendously and is influenced not only by intervening individuals with authority but also by pharmaceutical industry. Given immunotherapy especially with checkpoint inhibitors is being increasingly used for treatments of various cancers; its regulation and importation poses a constant challenge to developing countries. It is predicted that immunotherapies will replace majority of the cytotoxic chemotherapies in the near future for most of the cancers. Thereby, regulatory agencies of LMIC need to have dedicated staff for establishment of effective policies for rapid approval of essential cancer drugs.

Essential cancer drugs are often not available, not accessible, or not used appropriately in LMICs which is one of the greatest dilemmas of oncologic care [22]. Drug shortages are typically more common in LMICs and can lead to devastating outcomes in cancer patients [23]. This aspect of drug shortages is a critical, yet relatively neglected issue within the cancer management paradigm, and downstream the cost of cancer care can potentially increase tremendously. For example, if vincristine deficiency is sustained for few weeks or months, then it could result in a domino effect as this drug is the backbone of treatment of pediatric ALL, and if unavailable, can lead to multiple relapses, the treatment of which may be extremely complicated (including perhaps an allogeneic stem cell transplant) and expensive.

In 2011, the Council of International Pharmaceutical Federation called on "all stakeholders, including governments, pharmaceutical manufacturers, pharmacy wholesalers, pharmaceutical purchasing agencies, medicine insurance plans, pharmaceutical regulators and the pharmacy profession to urgently evaluate these issues and work to ensure continuity of medication supply so that the appropriate treatment of patients can be initiated and maintained". One of the solutions is to ensure smooth network of supply chain between the institutions that carry cancer drugs so that transfer can be ensued where the greatest need is apparent. Moreover, technologic advancements including machine learning algorithms (described below) can augment a smooth drug supply chain by not only prompting exchanges but also providing predictions for shortage of essential medications.

Pricing models that apply to the North American and European countries do not apply to the LMICs. Models where cost-sharing or cost-containment policies that can be enacted should be sought, and if not possible, then innovative strategies that can derive delivery of medications to the end users must happen. In India and Brazil, for some chemotherapy drugs, the pharmaceutical industry and the government have negotiated contracts to ensure cheaper drug availability to the cancer patients (subsidized cost versus on a governmental plan), and this includes local manufacturing for certain specialized medications. This is not an easy task, and would need to conform to the international patency laws; however, it is achievable as experienced by the abovementioned LMICs. Applications of generic medications and biosimilars should increase once equivalence in safety and efficacy is established.

Essential Need for a Safe and Effective Institutional Blood Bank

In many developing countries, it can be challenging to secure matched platelets and packed red blood cells in a timely fashion. This issue is complicated by the fact that some federal authorities in some countries restrict the blood banking and donor procedures to a central blood bank supervised by the government officials, and thus distribution can be at risk. This issue must be tackled before establishing a comprehensive cancer center, as many patients undergoing chemotherapy or stem cell transplantation require massive amounts of transfusion.

Applying Technologic Advancements in Oncology: Artificial Intelligence and Internet-of-Things

The technologic advancements are revolutionizing the cancer care especially with respect to diagnostics particularly in pathology and radiology [24]. The availability of big data has provided ample opportunity to evaluate and analyze predictive models in hematology [25, 26], medical oncology [27–29], and radiation oncology [30–32] via machine learning algorithms [33]. Apart from software development, the Internet-of-Things which runs on 5G network [34] is well posed to direct many aspects of healthcare including telehealth [35]. Some LMICs have already adapted these technology-based tools to improve the management of hematologic and oncologic management; though it requires initial investment in hardware/software technology and human resources, in long run, these technologies are predicted to lower cost of care and improve efficiencies. Thereby, we strongly propose to consider incorporation of technologic advancements in the current cancer framework going forward if possible and resources allow.

Unavailability of Specialized, but Essential Cancer Services: Radiotherapy and Stem Cell Transplantation

There are many services that are necessary for both curative and palliative management in cancers; however, due to expertise required, technology transfer issues, equipment infrastructure, and costs, they may be unavailable in LMICs. On the top of these essential services are stem cell transplantation (SCT) [15, 16] and radiotherapy [17–19]. These two services are necessary for many cancers and may be the only potential cure, and in order to achieve this cure, many patients from LMIC may travel outside their home country for the receipt of these services. One essential element of these services is that efforts must be concentrated to start with bare minimum requirements in order to establish at least one specialized unit, for example, for radiation therapy unit in a country, it is not essential to wait for funding and expertise for carbon-ion therapy or proton beam therapy, but can start with the cobalt therapy or with traditional linear accelerators. Similarly, for SCT, it is not imperative to have a huge infrastructure for allogeneic SCTs, when a center can start with the relatively low-risk autologous SCTs. Apart from getting expertise from outside the country for a new specialized program, one has to consider capacity building and skills training for physicians and nurses within a country.

Above, we mention some of the challenges and propose potential solutions for these issues pertaining to LMICs with respect to cancer care. It is apparent that one-size-fits-all solution is impractical and an approach tailored towards individualizing the priorities within a country given its resources is the most practical way of successfully implementing comprehensive cancer care.

Public Health Crises

Carcinogen Prevention

The tobacco epidemic due to a high prevalence of smoking has led to a much higher incidence of smoking-related cancers in the developing countries [36, 37]. While in the United States, the prevalence of smoking has decreased over the past few decades, in the developing countries, this trend has not been observed, and therefore, it is very likely that for the next few years there is a predictable increase in the incidence rates of cancers. Apart from cigarette smoking, certain behavioral practices are much more prevalent in the developing countries that also contribute to the increase in certain cancers in these populations which include betel nut (especially when mixed with slate lime) [38], herbal cigarettes [39], and shisha (pot smoking) [40].

Late Diagnosis

Due to either a lack of public health mandate for screening or non-implementation of policies of the screening programs, majority of the cancers are seen at a later-stage diagnosis.

Significant investment in the infrastructure for the above is needed. In the current era of media, the message also needs to get across to the public as well, and the media tools, for example, WhatsApp, Twitter, television, and direct-to-consumer messages could be tremendously helpful. Moreover, getting support by international organizations that have established programs for prevention and management of cancers should ideally be undertaken. Union for International Cancer Control (UICC) is one such nongovernmental organization that opens to membership to all developing and developed countries.

Conclusions

Above, we mention some of the challenges and propose potential solutions for these issues pertaining to LMICs with respect to cancer care. Some of the solutions are covered after each issue mentioned above. Some umbrella solutions include seeking funding by collaboration with charity and philanthropic organizations for financial and also in-kind support (patient transportation, housing, food, etc.). Holding fundraising events in collaboration with other government or private agencies could also be tremendously helpful.

It is apparent that one-size-fits-all solution is impractical and an approach tailored towards individualizing the priorities within a country given its resources is the most practical way of successfully implementing comprehensive cancer care.

Conflicts of Interest None of the authors declare any relevant COI.
Disclosures: SKH has received funding from Mallinckrodt, Pfizer, Novartis, Janssen.
SKH has received travel grants from MSD, Takeda, Gilead, and BMS.

References

1. Roser M, Ritchie H, Ortiz-Ospina E. World population growth. Our World in Data; 2013.
2. Kennedy BK, Berger SL, Brunet A, Campisi J, Cuervo AM, Epel ES, Franceschi C, Lithgow GJ, Morimoto RI, Pessin JE, Rando TA. Geroscience: linking aging to chronic disease. Cell. 2014;159(4):709–13.
3. Niccoli T, Partridge L. Ageing as a risk factor for disease. Curr Biol. 2012;22(17):R741–52.
4. Bellanger M, Zeinomar N, Tehranifar P, Terry MB. Are global breast cancer incidence and mortality patterns related to country-specific economic development and prevention strategies? J Global Oncol. 2018;4:1–16.

5. Torre LA, Bray F, Siegel RL, Ferlay J, Lortet-Tieulent J, Jemal A. Global cancer statistics, 2012. CA Cancer J Clin. 2015;65(2):87–108.
6. De Souza JA, Hunt B, Asirwa FC, Adebamowo C, Lopes G. Global health equity: cancer care outcome disparities in high-, middle-, and low-income countries. J Clin Oncol. 2016;34(1):6.
7. Navarro V, Muntaner C, Borrell C, Benach J, Quiroga Á, Rodríguez-Sanz M, Vergés N, Pasarín MI. Politics and health outcomes. Lancet. 2006;368(9540):1033–7.
8. https://seer.cancer.gov/about/. Accessed 07-07-2020.
9. Rochmyaningsih D. The developing world needs basic research too. Nature. 2016;534(7605):7–7.
10. Bosnjak Pasic M, Vidrih B, Sarac H, Pasic H, Vujevic L, Soldo Koruga A, Rajic F. Clinical trials in developing countries-ethical considerations. Psychiatr Danub. 2018;30(3):285–91.
11. Arabi YM, Al-Hameed F, Burns KE, Mehta S, Alsolamy SJ, Alshahrani MS, Mandourah Y, Almekhlafi GA, Almaani M, Al Bshabshe A, Finfer S. Adjunctive intermittent pneumatic compression for venous thromboprophylaxis. N Engl J Med. 2019;380(14):1305–15.
12. Jehan F, Nisar I, Kerai S, Balouch B, Brown N, Rahman N, Rizvi A, Shafiq Y, Zaidi AK. Randomized trial of amoxicillin for pneumonia in Pakistan. N Engl J Med. 2020;383(1):24–34.
13. Odedina FT, Shamley D, Okoye I, Ezeani A, Ndlovu N, Dei-Adomakoh Y, Meza K, Agaba R, Fathi P, Askins N. Landscape of oncology clinical trials in Africa. JCO Global Oncol. 2020;6:932–41.
14. Specchia ML, Frisicale EM, Carini E, Di Pilla A, Cappa D, Barbara A, Ricciardi W, Damiani G. The impact of tumor board on cancer care: evidence from an umbrella review. BMC Health Serv Res. 2020;20(1):73.
15. Hashmi SK, Srivastava A, Rasheed W, Adil S, Wu T, Jagasia M, Nassar A, Hwang WY, Hamidieh AA, Greinix HT, Pasquini MC. Cost and quality issues in establishing hematopoietic cell transplant program in developing countries. Hematol Oncol Stem Cell Ther. 2017;10(4):167–72.
16. Aljurf M, Weisdorf D, Hashmi SK, Nassar A, Gluckman E, Mohty M, Rizzo D, Pasquini M, Hamadani M, Saber W, Hari P. Worldwide Network for Blood and Marrow Transplantation (WBMT) recommendations for establishing a hematopoietic stem cell transplantation program in countries with limited resources (Part II): clinical, technical and socio-economic considerations. Hematol Oncol Stem Cell Ther. 2020;13(1):7–16.
17. Parkes J, Hess C, Burger H, Anacak Y, Ahern V, Howard SC, Elhassan M, et al. Recommendations for the treatment of children with radiotherapy in low-and middle-income countries (LMIC): a position paper from the Pediatric Radiation Oncology Society (PROS-LMIC) and Pediatric Oncology in Developing Countries (PODC) working groups of the International Society of Pediatric Oncology (SIOP). Pediatr Blood Cancer. 2017;64:e26903.
18. Datta NR, Samiei M, Bodis S. Radiation therapy infrastructure and human resources in low-and middle-income countries: present status and projections for 2020. Int J Radiat Oncol Biol Phys. 2014;89(3):448–57.
19. Abdel-Wahab M, Bourque JM, Pynda Y, Iżewska J, Van der Merwe D, Zubizarreta E, Rosenblatt E. Status of radiotherapy resources in Africa: an International Atomic Energy Agency analysis. Lancet Oncol. 2013;14(4):e168–75.
20. Price AJ, Ndom P, Atenguena E, Mambou Nouemssi JP, Ryder RW. Cancer care challenges in developing countries. Cancer. 2012;118(14):3627–35.
21. https://www.unhcr.org/figures-at-a-glance.html. Accessed 07-09-2020.
22. https://www.who.int/bulletin/volumes/85/4/06-033647/en/. Accessed July 10th, 2020.
23. Acosta A, Vanegas EP, Rovira J, Godman B, Bochenek T. Medicine shortages: gaps between countries and global perspectives. Front Pharmacol. 2019;10:763.
24. Savage N. How AI is improving cancer diagnostics. Nature. 2020;579(7800):S14.
25. Lee SI, Celik S, Logsdon BA, Lundberg SM, Martins TJ, Oehler VG, Estey EH, Miller CP, Chien S, Dai J, Saxena A. A machine learning approach to integrate big data for precision medicine in acute myeloid leukemia. Nat Commun. 2018;9(1):1–13.
26. Salah HT, Muhsen IN, Salama ME, Owaidah T, Hashmi SK. Machine learning applications in the diagnosis of leukemia: current trends and future directions. Int J Lab Hematol. 2019;41(6):717–25.

27. Yue W, Wang Z, Chen H, Payne A, Liu X. Machine learning with applications in breast cancer diagnosis and prognosis. Designs. 2018;2(2):13.
28. Wang H, Zhou Z, Li Y, Chen Z, Lu P, Wang W, Liu W, Yu L. Comparison of machine learning methods for classifying mediastinal lymph node metastasis of non-small cell lung cancer from 18 F-FDG PET/CT images. EJNMMI Res. 2017;7(1):11.
29. Manogaran G, Vijayakumar V, Varatharajan R, Kumar PM, Sundarasekar R, Hsu CH. Machine learning based big data processing framework for cancer diagnosis using hidden Markov model and GM clustering. Wirel Pers Commun. 2018;102(3):2099–116.
30. Shafai-Erfani G, Wang T, Lei Y, Tian S, Patel P, Jani AB, Curran WJ, Liu T, Yang X. Dose evaluation of MRI-based synthetic CT generated using a machine learning method for prostate cancer radiotherapy. Med Dosim. 2019;44(4):e64–70.
31. Giraud P, Giraud P, Gasnier A, El Ayachy R, Kreps S, Foy JP, Durdux C, Huguet F, Burgun A, Bibault JE. Radiomics and machine learning for radiotherapy in head and neck cancers. Front Oncol. 2019;9:174.
32. Valdes G, Solberg TD, Heskel M, Ungar L, Simone CB II. Using machine learning to predict radiation pneumonitis in patients with stage I non-small cell lung cancer treated with stereotactic body radiation therapy. Phys Med Biol. 2016;61(16):6105.
33. Chen B, Garmire L, Calvisi DF, Chua MS, Kelley RK, Chen X. Harnessing big 'omics' data and AI for drug discovery in hepatocellular carcinoma. Nat Rev Gastroenterol Hepatol. 2020;17:1–14.
34. Cheong IY, An SY, Cha WC, Rha MY, Kim ST, Chang DK, Hwang JH. Efficacy of mobile health care application and wearable device in improvement of physical performance in colorectal cancer patients undergoing chemotherapy. Clin Colorectal Cancer. 2018;17(2):e353–62.
35. Ray PP, Dash D, De D. A systematic review of wearable systems for cancer detection: current state and challenges. J Med Syst. 2017;41(11):180.
36. Islami F, Torre LA, Jemal A. Global trends of lung cancer mortality and smoking prevalence. Translat Lung Cancer Res. 2015;4(4):327.
37. Barta JA, et al. Global Epidemiology of Lung Cancer. Ann Glob Health. 2019;85(1):8, 1–16. https://doi.org/10.5334/aogh.2419.
38. https://www.who.int/mediacentre/news/releases/2003/priarc/en/#:~:text=A%20 CANCER%2DCAUSING%20HABIT&text=Areca%20nut%2C%20a%20common%20component%20of%20all%20betel%20quid%20preparations,itself%20is%20carcinogenic%20 to%20humans.
39. Gan Q, Yang J, Yang G, Goniewicz M, Benowitz NL, Glantz SA. Chinese "herbal" cigarettes are as carcinogenic and addictive as regular cigarettes. Cancer Epidemiol Prevent Biomark. 2009;18(12):3497–501.
40. Maziak W. The waterpipe: an emerging global risk for cancer. Cancer Epidemiol. 2013;37(1):1–4.

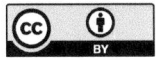

Index